Spiritual Care

Nursing Theory,
Research, and Practice

Spiritual Care
Nursing Theory,
Research, and Practice

Elizabeth Johnston Taylor, PhD, RN
Associate Professor
School of Nursing
Loma Linda University
Loma Linda, CA

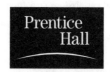

Prentice
Hall

Upper Saddle River, New Jersey 07458

Library of Congress Cataloging-in-Publication Data
Taylor, Elizabeth Johnston.
    Spiritual care : nursing theory, research, and
practice / by Elizabeth Johnston Taylor.
        p. ; cm.
    Includes bibliographical references.
    ISBN 0-13-028164-6
    1. Nursing—Religious aspects. 2. Nurse and
patient. 3. Spirituality. 4. Nursing—Psychological
aspects.
    [DNLM: 1. Nursing Care—psychology.
    2. Holistic Nursing—methods. 3. Nurse-Patient
    Relations. 4. Nursing Theory. 5. Religion and
    Medicine. WY 87 T239s 2002]
RT85.2 .T39 2002
610.73'01—dc21   2001021360

Notice: The author and the publisher of this volume have taken care that the information and recommendation contained herein are accurate at the time of publication. Nevertheless, it is difficult to ensure that all the information given is entirely accurate for all circumstances. The author and publisher disclaim any liabilities, loss, or damage incurred as a consequence, directly or indirectly, of the use and application of any of the contents of this volume.

Publisher: *Julie Alexander*
Executive Editor: *Maura Connor*
Acquisitions Editor: *Nancy Anselment*
Director of Production and Manufacturing: *Bruce Johnson*
Managing Production Editor: *Patrick Walsh*
Manufacturing Manager: *Ilene Sanford*
Production Liaison: *Julie Li*
Production Editor: *Linda Begley*
Creative Director: *Cheryl Asherman*
Cover Design Coordinator: *Maria Guglielmo*
Cover Designer: *Kevin Kall*
Editorial Consultant: *Patti Cleary*
Editorial Assistant: *Mary Ellen Ruitenberg*
Composition: *Rainbow Graphics*
Printing and Binding: *Von Hoffman Press*

Pearson Education LTD.
Pearson Education Australia PTY, Limited
Pearson Education Singapore, Pte. Ltd.
Pearson Education North Asia Ltd.
Pearson Education Canada, Ltd.
Pearson Educación de Mexico, S.A. de C.V.
Pearson Education—Japan
Pearson Education Malaysia, Pte. Ltd.
Pearson Education, Upper Saddle River, New Jersey

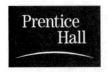

10 9 8 7 6 5 4 3 2 1
ISBN 0-13-028164-6

Dedication

To Lyndon Johnston Taylor . . .
My research assistant, technical support, and benefactor,
My best friend, my lover, and my husband
. . . a Godly man who inspires and inspirits me.

Contents

Preface

Spirituality in the context of health is reemerging in public and professional arenas as an essential and vital component of health care. As evidenced by mandates from national as well as local organizations, nurses are increasingly expected to incorporate the spiritual dimension within their care. Because spirituality represents an innate, integral dimension of all human beings, to nurse the whole client we must also nurse the spirit.

Nursing literature has addressed the topic of spirituality primarily in theoretical and conceptual terms, and its inability to offer practical guidance to support the provision of spiritual care has created a gap in our nursing knowledge. This text aims to fill this gap by providing practical guidance on many aspects of spiritual caregiving. Practice, however, must be supported by theory and research. The practice suggestions offered in this book follow from theory and research in nursing as well as other related disciplines.

Because of the deeply significant and often private nature of spirituality, communicating with clients about their spiritual needs requires sensitivity. Consideration of the role of the nurse with regards to spiritual matters raises important questions. Beyond offering the significant expertise of empathic listening and presencing, what role should the nurse play?

This text asserts that every nurse should strive to attain competence in the provision of sensitive, effective, and individualized spiritual care. To be effective, this care should incorporate the two-tiered approach to assessment presented in Chapter 5. If a spiritual need is identified during an initial, brief assessment (first tier), more extensive assessment follows (second tier). At any point, the nurse may conclude that a client does not require spiritual care, or requires it from a chaplain or other spiritual care expert. When referral is warranted, the client will still benefit from the nurse who provides the most basic spiritual care "interventions" of presencing and empathic listening.

For many clients, assessment will reveal some manifestation of spiritual need or the opportunity for enhancing spiritual well-being. These clients will benefit from nursing care that incorporates the spiritual care interventions presented in this book. This text presents varied approaches and a number of spiritual care interventions from which the nurse can select in order to address client needs. As with other areas of nursing practice, a nurse's ability to provide effective spiritual care will improve with practice.

An expression of spirituality, religion also is often a bridge to experiencing spirituality. Many nurses profess a religious orientation, which can enhance awareness of and sensitivity to client spiritual needs. The nurse's religious background may in some cases also create bias that can interfere with effective care. This text encourages the nurse to recognize that personal beliefs affect care and to develop and sustain awareness of personal beliefs in order to enhance the effectiveness of spiritual care. This text also embraces the position that nurses will derive significant benefits from engaging in activities that promote their own spiritual health.

Just as a scientific study is influenced by the context under which it is conducted, a book's approach will be influenced by the worldview of its author. The author, who has endeavored to present spirituality in a manner sensitive to diverse spiritual experiences, acknowledges a religio-cultural background that is Western and Judeo-Christian. Furthermore, the research and nursing literature available represents, for the most part, a similar framework. Sensitivity and appreciation for diversity can help to overcome limitations created by this or any other bias.

One way to show religio-cultural sensitivity is to refer to centuries as either being Before the Common Era (B.C.E.) or in the Common Era (C.E.), a generic way to refer to what Christians would consider anno Domini (A.D., or a year in the Christian era). This book, therefore, uses B.C.E. and C.E. to designate dates.

STRUCTURE OF THE TEXT

This text is organized into three sections. Part I explores spirituality in nursing in order to establish a basis for Part II, which addresses nursing practice issues and strategies that support spiritual caregiving, and Part III, which presents specific interventions for promoting client spiritual health.

Several features enhance learning about spiritual care. Boxes accompany the narrative to extend learning by synthesizing information and to illustrate concepts through examples such as case studies or nursing care plans. Research Profiles summarize studies and their relevance to practice. One Client's/Nurse's Story is a feature that illustrates the application of principles of spiritual care. Each chapter concludes with Key Points to support content review and Look Within to Learn questions to encourage the development of self-awareness. Highlighted references identify literature that is likely to be especially helpful to the reader who desires further knowledge.

Acknowledgments

Many individuals have shaped how the author views spirituality within the context of health care. Several have provided specific assistance to guide the preparation of this book. I am pleased to acknowledge these friends. I experience a profound sense of gratitude and happiness when I remember the gifts of:

Patti Cleary, an outstanding editorial consultant, whose writing expertise and conceptual creativity have significantly molded the contents of this text. Her practical guidance and skillful editing taught me much and made the book's birthing enjoyable.

Ministry experts Marsha Fowler, MS, MDiv, PhD, FAAN, Wil Alexander, MTh, PhD; my spiritual director Ann Morris; instructors at Centerpoint (Santa Barbara, California); and others who have instructed me about how to gently care for the spirit.

My students in "Spiritual Dimensions of Health" courses, my research informants, and persons for whom I have provided nursing care who have encouraged me to pursue this topic and taught me through their personal stories.

Content experts Richard Rice, MDiv, PhD (Chapter 7); Chaplains Larry VandeCreek, DMin, and David Girardin, MDiv, RN (Chapter 8); Robert Johnston, MDiv, PhD, and Siroj Sorajjakool, PhD (Chapter 10); and nurse reviewers whose critiques and encouragement strengthened these chapters.

Pre- and postdoctoral mentors Ruth McCorkle, PhD, FAAN, and Geraldine Padilla, PhD, who expertly taught me about theory and research.

Helen Emori King, PhD, RN, Dean of the Loma Linda University School of Nursing (Loma Linda, California), whose gracious support helped me to complete this project.

Nancy Anselment, Nursing Acquisitions Editor at Prentice Hall, whose work and vision recognized the need for this book and supported its creation.

Reviewers

The following reviewers provided valuable feedback during the writing process. We thank all these professionals for their contribution and attention to detail.

Norma E. Anderson RN-C, Ph.D.
Saint Louis University School of Nursing
Community Health
St. Louis, Missouri

Kathleen Blais Ed.D., RN
Florida International University
School of Nursing
North Miami, Florida

Barbara Mathews Blanton MSN, RN
Texas Woman's University
College of Nursing
Dallas, Texas

Janet Brown
California State University
School of Nursing
Chico, California

Lynn Keegan, RN, Ph.D., HNC, FAAN
Director, Holistic Nursing Consultants
Temple, Texas and Port Angeles, Washington

Rachel E. Spector, Ph.D., RN, CTN, FAAN
Boston College
Community Health
Chestnut Hill, Massachusetts

Spiritual Care
Nursing Theory,
Research, and Practice

Part I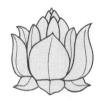

Exploring Spirituality in Nursing

1

What Is Spirituality?

Many aspects of spirituality are intangible, and the ways in which we humans experience spirituality can be highly individual. If you were to describe to a friend the taste of an exotic fruit, you might refer to it as sour enough to tease and sweet enough to please. You could add other descriptors like nutty, firm, robust, moist, or silky. Only after sampling the fruit, however, will your friend come to know how it tastes. And your friend's fruit-tasting experience may be very like—or very different from—your own.

Similarly, some aspects of spirituality are not easily described. Often, when people have what they define as a spiritual experience, they are unable to articulate it to their own satisfaction. Yet they are unwavering in their conviction that their experience has been spiritual.

Discussions about any concept, and in this case the concept of spirituality, benefit when the participants share at least to some degree an image of that concept. To establish common ground, this chapter explores various descriptions of spirituality and considers how spirituality is distinct from several related concepts. The chapter also reviews ways that spirituality can manifest among clients and how nurses perceive those manifestations.

DEFINING SPIRITUALITY

Consider how the word *spirit* is used in everyday conversation. Nurses sometimes describe clients as being in "good spirits," or as "highly spirited," or as possessing an "indomitable spirit." People may refer to others as having lost "their spirit" or their "will to live," or they may remark that someone's "spirits are at a low point."

Analysis of a concept typically examines dictionary definitions. Dictionaries define *spirituality* (synonymous with "spiritualness," according to the *Oxford English Dictionary*) by recognizing a number of possible meanings, including:

- Sacred
- Ecclesiastical (relating to a religious organization)
- Incorporeal (intangible or without a physical dimension)
- Moral (feelings or states of the soul)
- Holy or divine
- Of a pure essence
- Intellectual and higher endowments of the mind
- Highly refined in thought and feeling
- Spirited in the sense of witty or clever or volatile
- Spirits or supernatural entities (e.g., beings, ghosts)

Etymologically, the word *spirituality* shares the same root as words related to breathing (e.g., respiration, inspiration, expiration). These various meanings for the word suggest that for humans, spirituality represents a fundamental essence—a necessity—that energizes and guides action and thought.

Certain themes emerge in definitions of spirituality offered by a number of nurses who have written about spirituality. Dyson, Cobb, and Forman (1997) identified common themes as meaning, hope, relatedness/connectedness, beliefs/belief systems, and expressions of spirituality—dimensions of spirituality that nurses frequently identify. Dyson and colleagues also observed that nurses propose that these dimensions are found in the context of persons as they relate to self, others, or God. As Reed (1992) phrased it, spirituality involves intra-, inter-, and transpersonal relatedness.

Review of these definitions reveals spirituality to be a concept that applies to all persons. Spirituality is an innate, universal aspect of being human. Everyone has a spiritual dimension. This dimension integrates, motivates, energizes, and influences every aspect of a person's life. To illustrate how these themes are conveyed in definitions of spirituality, Box 1-1 offers a list selected from the nursing literature of the past three decades.

Box 1-1. Nursing Definitions of Spirituality

Vaillot (1970)   Spirituality is "the quality of those forces which activate us, or are the essential principle influencing us. Spiritual, although it might, does not necessarily mean religious; it also includes the psychological. The spiritual is opposed to the biological and mechanical, whose laws it may modify" (p. 30).

Colliton (1981)   Spirituality is "the life principle that pervades a person's entire being, including volitional, emotional, moral–ethical, intellectual, and physical dimensions, and generates a capacity for transcendent values" (p. 492).

Amenta (1986)   "The spiritual is the self, or I, the essence of personhood, the God within, that part which communes with the transcendent. It is that part of each individual which longs for ultimate awareness, meaning, value, purpose, beauty, dignity, relatedness, and integrity" (p. 117).

Stoll (1989)   Spirituality involves a vertical dimension (i.e., a person's relationship with God, the transcendent, supreme values) and a horizontal dimension (i.e., which "reflects and 'fleshes out' the supreme experiences of one's relationship with God through one's beliefs, values, life-style, quality of life, and interactions with self, others, and nature" (p. 7).

Reed (1992)   "Spirituality refers to the propensity to make meaning through a sense of relatedness to dimensions that transcend the self in such a way that empowers and does not devalue the individual. This relatedness may be experienced intrapersonally (as a connectedness within oneself), interpersonally (in the context of others and the natural

---

(continues)

Box 1-1. Nursing Definitions of Spirituality *(continued)*

	environment), and transpersonally (referring to a sense of relatedness to the unseen, God, or power greater than the self and ordinary resources)" (p. 350).
Fowler (cited in Fowler& Peterson, 1997)	"Spirituality is the way in which a person understands and lives life in view of her or his ultimate meaning, beliefs, and values. It is the unifying and integrative aspect of the person's life and, when lived intentionally, is experienced as a process of growth and maturity. It integrates, unifies, and vivifies the whole of a person's narrative or story, embeds his or her core identity, establishes the fundamental basis for the individual's relationship with others and with society, includes a sense of the transcendent, and is the interpretive lens through which the person sees the world. It is the basis for community for it is in spirituality that we experience our co-participation in the shared human condition. It may or may not be expressed or experienced in religious categories" (p. 47).
Narayanasamy (1999)	". . . is rooted in an awareness which is part of the biological make up of the human species. Spirituality is therefore present in all individuals and it may manifest as inner peace and strength derived from perceived relationship with a Transcendent God/an Ultimate Reality, or whatever an individual values as supreme. The spiritual dimension evokes feelings which demonstrate the existence of love, faith, hope, trust, awe, and inspirations; therein providing meaning and a reason for existence" (pp. 274–275).
Dossey & Guzzetta (2000)	"a unifying force of a person; the essence of being that permeates all of life and is manifested in one's being, knowing, and doing; the interconnectedness with self, others, nature, and God/Life Force/Absolute/Transcendent" (p. 7).

Discussions of spirituality within nursing have evolved over time, influenced by the philosophies of holism and humanism (Emblen, 1992). Prior to the 1970s, nurses tended to use the term *religion* when discussing spirituality. With the increasing secularization of our society, nurses have recognized the need to distinguish religiosity from spirituality. It is the broader, encompassing concept of spirituality in which nurses now tend to be interested. Another term that some nurses have taken care with defining is the term *God* (Dyson et al., 1997). For example, Stoll (1989) clearly introduces the term *God* with the caveat "as defined by that person." Others attempt to avoid "God" language by using terms such as higher power, supreme being, or Ultimate Other. Some recognize "supreme values" instead of a deity.

Concepts are "words or [a] collection of words expressing a mental image of some phenomenon" (Fawcett & Downs, 1992, p. 16). Concepts in nursing literature that express aspects of spirituality include:

- **Inspiriting** has been defined as "the unfolding mystery through harmonious interconnectedness that springs from inner strength" (Burkhardt, 1989, p. 72). Burkhardt borrowed this term from Jourard (1964) who suggested that life events can be inspiriting or dispiriting. Jourard proposed that how people respond to life events, that is, whether they become inspirited (uplifted) or dispirited (disheartened), determines their "spirit titre."
- **Spiritual quality of life** is a phrase used by some researchers who recognize spirituality to be one dimension of quality of life or well-being. For example, McMillan's Hospice Quality of Life Index (McMillan & Weitzner, 2000) explores the meaningfulness of life and relationship with God in order to measure spiritual quality of life. The City of Hope quality-of-life model (Ferrell et al., 1996) suggests that strengthened belief, hope, religiosity, and inner strength are components of spiritual well-being.
- **Spiritual well-being** is a construct found frequently in nursing literature (e.g., Hood Morris, 1996; Reed, 1992). Poloutzian and Ellison's Spiritual Well-Being Scale (Ellison, 1983), used by many nurse researchers, is composed of existential (i.e., pertaining to issues of the meaning of life) and religious well-being subscales. After reviewing research and theoretical discussions about spirituality, Hood Morris (1996) identified harmonious interconnectedness, creative energy, and faith in a power greater than oneself as the key attributes of spiritual well-being.

- **Spiritual disequilibrium**, a phrase coined by Dombeck (1996), describes the state of inner chaos that results when a client's most cherished beliefs are challenged. For example, when diagnosis of a life-threatening illness causes someone to question previously held assumptions about self-worth or the love and fairness of God, he or she may experience spiritual disequilibrium.
- **Spiritual need, problem, and concern** are terms used frequently in nursing literature to address aspects of spiritual caregiving (e.g., Highfield & Cason, 1983; Amenta, 1986). Stoll (1983) defined spiritual needs as "any factor(s) necessary to establish and/or maintain one's relationship to God, as defined by that person" (p. 577).
- **Spiritual distress** is terminology that is incorporated within nursing diagnoses that address spirituality. Kim, McFarland, and McLane (1991) defined spiritual distress as the "disruption in the life principle that pervades a person's entire being and that integrates and transcends one's biological and psychosocial nature" (p. 63). Hood Morris (1996) argued that spiritual distress can foster spiritual growth as well as spiritual well-being.
- **Spiritual pain; spiritual alienation; and spiritual anxiety, guilt, anger, loss,** and **despair** were identified by O'Brien (1999) as nursing diagnoses related to "alterations in spiritual integrity." The most frequent of these diagnoses, spiritual pain, was defined by O'Brien as "an individual's perception of hurt or suffering associated with that part of his or her person that seeks to transcend the realm of the material; it is manifested by a deep sense of hurt stemming from feelings of loss or separation from one's God or deity, a sense of personal inadequacy or sinfulness before God and man; or a pervasive condition of loneliness of spirit" (p. 71).
- **Spiritual perspective** was defined by a team of researchers who analyzed concepts related to spirituality as the "integrating and creative energy based on belief in, and a feeling of interconnectedness with, a power greater than self" (Haase, Britt, Coward, Leidy, & Penn, 1992, p. 143).

No nurse author has yet analyzed how each of these concepts overlaps or is related. The questions arise: Is spiritual perspective similar to inspiritedness? Is spiritual well-being the same as spiritual quality of life? Do spiritual distress and pain represent the negative end of a spiritual need or problem continuum (assuming that spiritual needs or problems can include positive needs [e.g., the need to express joy after the birth of a child])?

Several nurses have, however, systematically analyzed the concept of spirituality or related aspects (e.g., Burkhardt, 1989; Emblen, 1992; Goldberg, 1998; Haase et al., 1992; Hood Morris, 1996; Mansen, 1993). The method typically utilized to critically explore and refine the concept of spirituality is concept analysis. This process of analyzing a concept directs the inquirer to first consider all the possible uses, definitions, and meanings of a concept, to identify antecedents and consequences of the concept, and to distinguish and refine the concept by comparing it with related or contrary concepts. Box 1-2 presents an example of a concept analysis.

Although the language used to discuss spirituality varies, nurses have made great strides recently at using an analytical process to conceptualize spirituality. This process will no doubt continue to bring refinement and clarity to discussions about the nature of spirituality. Some argue, however, that achieving a unified definition of spirituality may be inap-

---

Box 1-2. Research Profile: "Connection: An Exploration of Spirituality in Nursing" by Goldberg (1998)

Purpose: To explore the meaning of the concept spirituality as it relates to nursing care, by discovering new dimensions of the concept of spirituality and looking for similarities and differences among spirituality and related concepts.

Method: Walker and Avant's approach to concept synthesis (i.e., extensive literature review to identify new dimensions of an old concept, looking for similarities and discrepancies among related concepts). The author then sorts these dimensions into categories and applies a unifying label to the concepts.

Main Findings: Primary phenomena related to spirituality identified in nursing literature were meaning, presencing, empathy and compassion, giving hope, love, religion and transcendence, touch and healing. *Connection* represents all these phenomena. Author implies that nurse clinicians have a more narrow perception of what spiritual care entails, whereas they easily recognized that "connection" with clients can have many facets. Spiritual care is "inseparable" from other dimensions of nursing care because spirit motivates the body.

Nursing Implications: Quality nursing care requires excellent interpersonal skills and adequate time and resources for providing spiritual care.

propriate, especially considering the mysterious and metaphysical nature of the concept (McSherry & Draper, 1998). Yet Emblen (1992) concluded that a common understanding of spirituality will assist nurses to communicate clearly with each other about spiritual care, and in turn will foster spiritual caregiving.

RELATED CONCEPTS: DISTINCTIONS AND CONNECTIONS

An issue raised often by nurses is the distinction between spirituality and other aspects of human nature, especially how spirituality differs from religiosity. Nurses seek to understand how to distinguish the spiritual dimension from the psychological or emotional and to appreciate how ethics, culture, and spirituality are related. An overview of concepts related to but distinct from spirituality will help to clarify the nature of spirituality and spiritual care.

Religion

A dictionary of religion defines *religion* as "a system of beliefs and practices that are relative to superhuman beings . . . beings who can do things ordinary mortals cannot do" (Smith, 1995, p. 893). Pargament (1997) defined religion quite differently, as "a search for significance in ways related to the sacred" (p. 32). Whether or not a person's religion is of an organized form, religion offers a participant a specific worldview and answers to questions about ultimate meaning. Religion can also offer guidance about how to live harmoniously with self, others, nature, and god(s). This direction is presented through a religion's belief system (e.g., its myths, doctrines, stories, dogma), and is acknowledged when one participates in rituals or other religious practices and observances.

From these definitions of religion, it is evident that religion is a narrower concept than spirituality. Remember, spirituality refers to that part of being human that seeks meaningfulness through intra-, inter-, and transpersonal connection (Reed, 1992). That is, people strive for a sense of meaningfulness, and they do so by being at peace, in harmony—inwardly, with other people and nature, and with that which they see as the Ultimate Other. Religion can be seen as a bridge to spirituality in that it encourages ways of thinking, feeling, and behaving that help people to experience this sense of meaningfulness. Religious practice is also a way for individuals, often in the context of sharing a similar orientation with others, to express their spirituality. Expressions of spirituality, however, are not restricted to religious practice. It is important to recognize that human beings, however they choose to express their spirituality, are spiritual beings. Even those who may see themselves as not religious will, as all humans do, seek meaning. Thus, spirituality, a component of being human, is a broader concept than religion, which is practiced by many but not all humans.

Psychological Dimension

Because the physical, psychological, and spiritual are integrated, interacting dimensions of whole persons, a distinction between the spiritual and psychological dimensions is an abstract and artificial separation. It is, nevertheless, a useful distinction to make for purposes of assessment and treatment (Highfield & Cason, 1983; Mansen, 1993). Nurses can avoid misinterpreting spiritual needs for psychosocial needs if they are aware of this distinction. Spilka, Spangler, and Nelson (1983) contrasted these two dimensions by suggesting that the psychological dimension referred to issues of human relationships on an immediate level (e.g., dealing with grief, loss, emotional and physical pain), whereas the spiritual dimension referred to "issues of life in terms of ultimate meanings, values, relationships with the Ultimate" (p. 99).

An analogy cited by Stallwood and Stoll (1975) may offer the best way of understanding how these dimensions interact: Considering a light-bulb analogous to a human, think of the glass, aluminum, and other tangible materials that comprise it as representing the physical dimension; think of the light and warmth the bulb elicits as the psychological; and the electrical current that energizes and ultimately provides the meaning and function for the bulb as the spiritual dimension.

Stoll (1989) differentiates the spiritual from the physical and psychosocial dimensions by positing that the spiritual aspect of being human allows for awareness and feeling of connection to deity or supreme values. The physical is what allows a person to experience—to taste, see, hear, smell, feel, and to be experienced by others. The emotions, intellect, will, and moral sense contribute to personality and identity and comprise the psychosocial dimension. To summarize Stoll's perspective:

- The physical dimension is world-consciousness.
- The psychosocial dimension is self-consciousness and self-identity.
- The spiritual dimension is God-consciousness or relatedness to a deity or supreme values.

Culture

Culture is often inappropriately equated with ethnicity. A broad definition of *culture* will recognize that it is the various ways of living and thinking that are built up and shared by a particular group of people (Leininger, 1988; Martsolf, 1997). A specific culture will share similar values, norms, lifestyles, rules, language, and beliefs. Beliefs can arise from a sense of spirituality or from one's cultural affiliation, and therefore spirituality and culture can overlap or be difficult to separate. Martsolf (1997) suggested three ways in which spirituality and culture can be related:

1. Spirituality can be determined entirely by culture.
2. Spirituality can be determined by life experiences unrelated to culture.
3. Spirituality can be influenced by both culture and personal experiences that are in opposition to the cultural norm.

Religion, an expression of or a bridge to spirituality, frequently is shared within a group and therefore can become a culture itself. The Amish people, many of whom reside in Pennsylvania and Indiana, share a religion that influences them to live in aggregates. They practice customs of simplicity, for example, working as farmers, avoiding technology, and wearing plain dress, that illustrate the interrelationship of spirituality, religion, and culture.

To determine how culture may relate to a client's spiritual responses to illness, researchers have investigated aspects of spirituality and religiousness among culturally diverse people. Some nurse researchers, in studying culture and ethnicity's impact on client adjustment to illness, have observed that religiosity and spiritual beliefs play a significant role in how clients interpret and make sense of their illness, and in how they cope with it. For example, spiritual beliefs and faith have been observed to influence and predict health-related quality of life (HRQOL) among Hispanics and African Americans living with cancer (Juarez, Ferrell, & Borneman, 1998; Wan et al., 1999).

Other research has explored how ill persons (especially those with cancer) from the different major ethnic groups utilize complementary therapies, including spiritual practices. Several studies document that Hispanic Americans and African Americans are more likely than Asian Americans and European Americans to use prayer, meditation, and other spiritual healing practices (Cushman, Wade, Factor-Litvak, Kronenberg, & Firester, 1999; Higgins & Learn, 1999; Lee, Lin, Wrensch, Adler, & Eisenberg, 2000; Potts, 1996). Likewise, persons of these two ethnic groups are more likely to perceive their spirituality as an important part of healthful living and will be more likely to identify a spiritual need and want help with it when they are sick. Interestingly, research conducted by Moadel and colleagues (1999), found ethnicity to be the best predictor of high spiritual need among cancer patients.

Morality and Ethics

Ethics guides the determination of what is "right" and "wrong" and deals with "oughts" and "shoulds." Morality refers to the rules a society has created for promoting ethical conduct, or right and virtuous behavior. Considering that spirituality by definition recognizes individual needs for meaning and concern about supreme values, it certainly can be related to morality and ethics. Applying values and assigning meaning to things in life is inherent in ethical and moral decision making. And the acts of valuing and finding meaning are acts involving and reflecting spirituality. When one asks ethical questions (e.g., "What is right in this situation? What ought I to do?"), one is also inevitably raising spiritual questions (e.g., "What is the source of truth for me?").

One Nurse's Story (see Box 1-3), presents a first-person account that illustrates the interrelationship of spiritual, religious, psychosocial/emotional, cultural, and ethical dimensions.

Box 1-3. One Nurse's Story: The Interrelatedness of Human Dimensions

Background
Joy Tan, a 20-year-old Chinese American nursing student, lives in a large U.S. metropolitan area. She and her parents had lived in the United States for nearly seven years when she wrote the following description of her spirituality:

My family's religion and culture has had a major influence on my spirituality. Because I was raised in an Asian culture, I continue to have a lot of Asian characteristics. For example, I am very shy, quiet, and family oriented. My mom raised me and she has a strong influence on my religion and spirituality. My mom believes in Buddhism and has certain beliefs about romantic love (i.e., the importance of being a virgin

(continues)

Box 1-3. One Nurse's Story: The Interrelatedness of Human Dimensions *(continued)*

before marriage and arranged marriage). However, I think that although virginity is important, I don't believe marriages should be arranged. I think that marriage should be between two persons who are in love.

Since I was a child, my mom told my brother and me to pray to the Buddha for protection from harm and for a better education. One of my childhood memories is of my mom taking us to the temple. Another is of burning incense to the Buddha at home. I had no idea what it meant to give incense at the time; I just did it because my mom said to. All I cared about was eating the delicious fruits and Chinese cookies that were offered to the Buddha, which can be eaten after the prayers. But now I know what giving incense means; it means to pray to the Buddha for protection or to ask for something.

I was taught by mom to be a moral person. To me, being moral means being honest, not lying, and not cheating. These are also the basic principles of Buddhism. My spirituality embraces many, but not all, the principles of Buddhism. For example, I don't believe one has to be a vegetarian, not smoke or drink alcohol. I do believe that the Buddha will help anyone who truly and sincerely believes in the existence of Buddha.

Now that I have become an adult, I lack the dedication and commitment to my Buddhist worship practices. The daily tasks of everyday living have taken me away from my prayers. I do still believe in Buddha, and I give incense to him on Chinese holidays. I believe that as long as one is sincere and truly believes in the existence of the Buddha, he will hear one's prayers.

Being a moral person gives meaning to my life. I believe that this is how one should live life. People should live life in such a way that when they get old, they can look back on life and have no regrets. Doing anything that goes against the basic principles of Buddha would be bad and regrettable. In this way, I think my religion and spirituality have a positive effect on me; they guide me toward a moral life.

I have matured spiritually during my life. For example, while I used to pray just because my mom told me to, now I pray because I

**Box 1-3. One Nurse's Story: The Interrelatedness
of Human Dimensions** *(concluded)*

---

believe. I had an experience three years ago that caused me to feel
very angry and depressed. I even tried to kill myself. I prayed to the
Buddha every day in a very sincere way, and I finally got my wish.
This made me think that Buddha was moved by my hurt. From then
on, I have really believed in the Buddha. When my wish finally came
true, I had a change of heart. I now realize, as I look back, that this
was just a stage in my life that I needed to accept, learn, and grow
from. Now when I am faced with obstacles in my life, I just think of
them as transitions and remember that the experience will only make
me stronger.

Analysis
Joy's description reveals how a person's spirituality relates to his or
her experience of religion and culture and influences one's psychosocial state, ethics, and morality. The religious philosophy of
Buddhism has influenced how Joy thinks about a transcendent
being (i.e., she worships the Buddha whom she views as powerful
and sensitive to her needs), how she relates to suffering (e.g., she
prays when depressed), and how she lives and relates to others
every day (e.g., chooses to remain a virgin until marriage). Joy's
religion also influences her morality and ethics. Her Buddhist
beliefs help her to decide what is right and wrong and what her values are, and guide her in living morally. Joy also states that living a
moral life gives her meaningfulness (which most consider to be an
element of spiritual well-being).

Joy's Asian cultural background is intertwined with her religious
beliefs. Joy's worship practices are culturally influenced (e.g., Joy is
reminded to pray on Chinese holidays). Psychosocial/emotional struggles prompt Joy, who prayed when she felt suicidal to draw on spiritual resources. Although she does not explicitly indicate this, it is
likely that prayer and the inner sense that she is living what she
believes to be an ethical lifestyle contribute to her sense of psychosocial or emotional well-being.

MANIFESTATIONS OF SPIRITUALITY

The definitions of spirituality reviewed above provide an abstract and broad view of the concept. But how does spiritual well-being or distress manifest? How will nurses know it when they see it? Some examples of how spirituality manifests may be beneficial to the reader at this point. (For additional information on of the various dimensions of spirituality, see Chapter 5.)

Some have suggested that spirituality manifests itself at different levels (Koenig & Pritchett, 1998; Nolan & Crawford, 1997; Reed, 1992). That is, spirituality manifests in how:

- A person relates to self
- A person relates to others
- A person relates to that which is transcendent (i.e., that which is beyond, above, ultimate, or supreme)
- Groups of people relate among and within themselves

Aspects of a person's spirituality become recognizable when a spiritual need emerges. Spiritual needs can result from distressful experiences. The physiological and emotional experience of stress is not limited to negative experiences. Eustress, a type of stress that one experiences in response to positive events, can also trigger spiritual needs.

Examples of individual spiritual needs may include the need to have purpose, to have hope, to express feelings (of gladness or sadness), to transcend challenges, to be thankful, and so forth. The desire to relate to and worship an Ultimate Other are also spiritual needs for individuals. Spiritual needs at the interpersonal level include the desire to forgive and be forgiven and to love and be loved by others. Nolan and Crawford (1997) suggest that groups have spiritual needs, too. For example, groups need to contribute positively to their world and perceive that their contribution is valued.

Awareness of these common ways in which spirituality may evidence or express itself among clients is requisite to providing spiritual care. In fact, because all humans have a spiritual dimension, all clients in some way will express and manifest their spirituality to nurses. Nurses often fail to recognize and appreciate these expressions of the spiritual nature and therefore fail to address this dimension (Highfield & Cason, 1983; McSherry, 1998). Box 1-4 shows how spiritual needs may manifest at different levels and without being expressed in religious language.

Box 1-4. Manifestations of Spirituality: Common Spiritual Needs		
Category of Spiritual Need	**Examples of Spiritual Needs**	**Illustrative Statements or Behaviors**
Needs related the to self	Need for meaning and purpose	"Sometimes I wonder what purpose of my life is."
	Need to feel useful	"No one needs me anymore, it seems."
	Need for vision	"It's hard to think that there is anything more I can contribute to this world."
	Need for hope	"I feel desperate—nothing can help me overcome my problem."
	Need for support in coping with life transitions	"I realize how important it is now for me to have my friends and loved ones helping me."
	Need to adapt to increasing dependency	"I don't want my family to have to take care of me when I'm old."
	Need to transcend life challenges	"I wish I could find a silver lining in all my problems."
	Need for personal dignity	"I wish the staff would respect my privacy more."

(continues)

Box 1-4. Manifestations of Spirituality: Common Spiritual Needs *(continued)*		

	Need to express feelings	"Ha! Who wants to listen to me?"
	Need to be thankful	"Feeling grateful makes me feel better."
	Need to accept and prepare for death	"I'm afraid to die."
	Need to fellowship with others	"I miss being able to go to my support group every week."
	Need to love and serve others	"I try to help others who like me are coping with breast cancer."
	Need to confess and be forgiven	"I wish I could tell my dad how sorry I am about what I did to him."
	Need for continuity with the past	"Praying to my grandma makes me feel better." (Or making a scrapbook, studying personal genealogy, or reminiscing).
Needs related to others	Need to forgive others	"I feel so betrayed; and I know my anger is eating me inside."
	Need to cope with loss of loved ones	"I miss my loved one so much; I can't live without him/her."

Box 1-4. Manifestations of Spirituality: Common Spiritual Needs *(continued)*

Needs related to the Transcedant	Need to be certain there is a God or Ultimate Power in Universe	"How can anyone be absolutely sure there is some guiding force running this world?"
	Need to believe that God is loving	"Because of all the bad stuff that has happened to me, I wonder if God is loving or if He loves me."
	Need to experience God as present	"I wish I could feel God more personally—like a friend."
	Need to serve and worship God	"Going to synagogue and keeping mitzvah allow me to return love to God."
	Need to learn from Scripture or other sources considered inspired by God	"I like to read my Bible every day; it helps me to understand the world."
Needs among and within groups	Need to contribute to the improvement of one's community	A business club that raises funds for a school.
	Need to recognize the power for positive change that groups of individuals can make	"Individually, I can do a little to better the world; collectively, we can do a lot to change the world."

(continues)

Box 1-4. Manifestations of Spirituality: Common Spiritual Needs
(concluded)

	Need to understand duties and responsibilities	A service organization that modifies its vision and mission to meet the needs of a community
	Need to be respected and valued	A sociocultural group of persons (e.g., impoverished, disabled, Latinos, Haitians) who unify to demand better treatment from those who oppress them.
	Achievement of personal growth of members of group	A religious organization that fosters spiritual growth of its members
	Knowing what and when to give and take	A nature club that strives to preserve natural habitat or a prayer group that prays for its community and leaders

Sources: Koenig, H., & Pritchett, J. (1998). Religion and psychotherapy. In H. Koenig (Ed.), *Handbook of religion and mental health* (Chapter 22). San Diego, CA: Academic Press; and Nolan, P., & Crawford, P. (1997). Towards a rhetoric of spirituality in mental health care. *Journal of Advanced Nursing, 26,* 289–294.

When Taylor, Highfield, and Amenta (1994) surveyed oncology nurse clinicians about how they perceived spiritual needs to manifest themselves among their clients, the nurses identified a broad range of indicators. More than half of the behaviors they reported were not overt expressions of spiritual need. While these nurses did identify overt indicators (such as mentioning God, faith, or the search for meaning or expressing hopelessness or guilt), they also identified more subtle expressions of spiritual need (e.g., anxiety, anger, crying). These indicators of spiritual need also are similar to "defining characteristics" that indicate a nursing diagnosis of spiritual distress (see Chapter 6). No list could be complete, however, considering the complexity and variability of people—and of their spiritual dimensions.

Although it is valuable to know which needs nurses identify as spiritual, it is perhaps more important to understand how clients characterize their spiritual needs. Nurse researchers who have explored spiritual needs as identified by clients include Emblen and Halstead (1993); Hermann (2001); Fitchett, Burton, and Sivan (1997). Fitchett and colleagues indicate that the most frequently reported spiritual needs of 101 inpatient psychiatric and medical/surgical clients were:

- To receive care and support
- To experience God's presence
- To have opportunities to pray
- To gain a sense of purpose and meaning in life
- To receive visits from and engage in prayer with a chaplain

It is important to note that over three-quarters of these clients reported that they were aware of at least three spiritual needs during their hospitalization. Other studies identify additional spiritual needs, including the need to:

- Talk about spiritual issues
- Feel peaceful and comforted
- Experience nature
- Laugh and think happy thoughts
- Resolve bitter feelings
- See others smile
- Be with friends, family, and children
- Enjoy inspirational readings, music, and thoughts

SPIRITUAL DEVELOPMENT

Just as individuals develop physically, cognitively, and morally, they also develop spiritually. Several theologians have identified specific linear stages that individuals may progress through while maturing spiritually.

However, because Fowler's (1981) stages of faith development are the most frequently cited, they will be reviewed here. Although the term *faith* typically implies religious faith, Fowler recognized faith as a universal human phenomenon that leads persons to need and find meaning, an understanding of themselves in relation to their world. Fowler arrived at these seven stages of faith development after analyzing in-depth interviews with over 400 individuals who ranged in age from 3–84 years.

1. *Undifferentiated faith* is the label given to the period of infancy to three years when neonates and toddlers are acquiring the fundamental spiritual qualities of trust and mutuality, as well as courage, hope, and love. The transition to the next stage of faith begins when the child's language and thought start to converge, allowing for the use of symbolism. Sadly, it is also possible that these spiritual qualities can be undermined, rather than developed. This occurs, for an extreme example, when a parent consistently abuses a baby or toddler.

2. *Intuitive–Projective faith* is observable among children 3 to 7 years of age. This is the "fantasy-filled, imitative phase in which the child can be powerfully and permanently influenced by examples, moods, actions and stories of the visible faith" (p. 133). During this stage, children relate intuitively to the ultimate conditions of existence through stories and images, the fusion of facts and feelings. What is make-believe or magically concocted is what is reality. For a child in this stage of faith, for example, Santa Claus is real and God may be viewed literally as a big, smiling (or frowning) granddaddy in the sky (depending on the stories the important adults in the child's life tell).

3. *Mythic–Literal faith* is found among school-aged children (up to 12 years) but can linger even into adulthood. During this stage of faith, children are attempting to sort out what is fantasy from what is fact, by demanding proofs or demonstrations of reality. Stories become a critically important means for children this age to find meaning and to give organization to experience. It is a task of these children to learn not only the stories but the beliefs and practices of their community. They accept stories and beliefs literally rather than with abstract meanings. In this stage, for example, a Latter Day Saints child will begin learning the stories of the Bible and Book of Mormon, accepting them at face value; these stories will provide the child with a way of making sense of the community and the world of which he or she is a part.

4. When a child (or adolescent) begins to reflect on the incongruities observed between stories, the transition to the *Synthetic–Conventional faith* stage begins. This stage of faith usually applies to adolescents and teens, but can characterize some adults. The stage of faith accompanies the individual's experience of the world that is now beyond the family unit (e.g., school, media), and must provide a helpful understanding of this extended environment. While faith "must synthesize values and information; it must provide a basis for identity and outlook" (p. 172). At this stage, individuals generally conform to the beliefs of those around them, because they have not yet reflected or studied these beliefs objectively. Thus, beliefs and values of teens are often held tacitly. For example, an adolescent or teen raised by observant Jews will likely continue to observe the Jewish practices of parents and accept parents' beliefs.

5. *Individuative–Reflective faith* is typically observed among young adults, but may continue into later adulthood. This stage of faith is characterized by the development of a self-identity and worldview that is differentiated from those of others. The individual forms independent commitments, lifestyle, beliefs, and attitudes. The child who obediently attended mom's Roman Catholic mass every Sunday will now examine independently what religious practices and beliefs to accept. Another characteristic of this stage of development is the demythologizing of symbols into conceptual meanings. To illustrate, the young adult who was taught as a child not to place anything on top of holy scriptures because of their sacredness now understands that this is not religious edict, but rather an authority's attempt to teach respect for an object that informs the reader about what is sacred.

6. *Conjunctive faith* usually is found among adults past midlife. At this stage, adults find new appreciation for their past, value their inner voices, and become aware of deep-seated myths, prejudices, and images that are indwelling because of their social background. An individual with conjunctive faith "strives to unify opposites in mind and experience" and allows "vulnerability to the strange truths of those who are 'other' " (p. 198). For example, instead of trying to dissuade or avoid another with differing spiritual beliefs, a person in this stage of faith would embrace persons of other faith traditions, recognizing that in their faith may be new understanding. Also, an adult whose faith is conjunctive may practice prayer in a way that allows listening to the deeper self, instead of petitionary praying.

7. The *Universalizing* stage of faith is infrequently reached. Those in this stage of faith have a "sense of an ultimate environment [that] is inclusive of all being. They have become incarnators and actualizers of the spirit of an inclusive and fulfilled human community" (p. 200). These persons work to unshackle social, political, economic, or ideological burdens in society. They fully love life, yet simultaneously hold it loosely. Fowler identified Martin Luther King, Mahatma Gandhi, and Mother Teresa as examples of those having developed this level of faith.

SPIRITUAL CARE: NURSING IMPLICATIONS

Of central importance to this book is spiritual care. Few explicit definitions exist for this construct. Mayer (1992; with credit to Didomizio [1983]) suggested that spiritual care be defined as "the style by which the nurse integrates all aspects of care for the patient" (p. 37). That is, because spirituality is an integrative factor that connects all aspects of a person's life, nursing care is most effective when it acknowledges this integration.

Taylor, Amenta, and Highfield (1995) offered the following definition for spiritual care: "the health-promoting attendance to responses to stress that have an impact on an individual's or group's spiritual perspective" (p. 31). Simply put, the purpose of spiritual nursing care is to facilitate spiritual health. A common expression, "boosting someone's spirits," captures some aspects of the essence of spiritual care. In this book, we will define spiritual care as the activities and ways of being that bring spiritual quality of life, well-being, and function—all of which are dimensions of health—to clients.

Responses of oncology nurse clinicians to a survey asking them to define spiritual care reveals that many nurses equate spiritual care with overall effective nursing care (Taylor, Amenta, & Highfield, 1995). They most frequently described spiritual care as holistic, promoting well-being by nurturing or comforting the body, mind, and spirit, or providing overall good nursing care. As respondents phrased it, "Nurses do [support a client's spirit] all the time when they provide care in thoughtful, respectful ways. It may be as simple as meeting the practical needs of the patient with a loving and caring heart." Bedside nurses, however, often define spiritual care in concrete and practical terms, often focusing on specific measures to provide spiritual care (e.g., facilitating relationships and religious practices; promoting meaning, hope, love, and other spiritual qualities). Some suggest that who a nurse is as a person influences the provision of spiritual care (e.g., "being there," being respectful, and being willing to share personal beliefs).

In addition to reviewing definitions of the central concepts of spiritu- *nurse*
ality and spiritual care, it is necessary to recognize the underlying assump- *assump-*
tions nurses hold about spiritual care because these assumptions deter- *tion*
mine if and how care is provided. A total of 31 assumptions and principles
about spiritual care for clients, their families, professional caregivers,
communities, research, and education were identified by the Spirituality
Work Group of the International Work Group on Death, Dying, and
Bereavement (1990). These assumptions acknowledge that everyone has a
spiritual dimension that is expressed in various ways and influences how
clients and their caregivers experience illness, dying, or bereavement.

Because clients are sometimes unable to talk about their spiritual
needs, the Spirituality Work Group's principles encourage health care professionals to address spiritual concerns with sensitivity in order to support
disclosure. They also advocate providing care, conducting research, and
promoting education that fosters spiritual growth. Box 1-5 explores further
these assumptions about and principles to guide spiritual care. Although
nurses who care for the terminally ill may hold these assumptions, the
degree to which all nurses accept them is a subject for further research.

Box 1-5. Selected Assumptions and Principles of Spiritual Care	
Assumption	**Principle**
Each person has a spiritual dimension.	In the total care of a person, his or her spiritual nature must be considered along with the mental, emotional, and physical dimensions.
In a multicultural society, a person's spiritual nature is expressed in religious and philosophical beliefs and practices that differ widely depending on one's race, gender, social status, religion, ethnicity, and experience.	No single approach to spiritual care is satisfactory for all in a multicultural society; many kinds of resources are needed.

(continues)

Box 1-5. Selected Assumptions and Principles of Spiritual Care (*continued*)

Spirituality has many facets. It is expressed and enhanced in formal and informal ways, religious and secular ways.	A broad range of opportunities for expressing and enhancing one's spirituality should be available and accessible.
The environment shapes and can enhance or diminish one's spirituality.	Care should be taken to offer settings that will accommodate individual preference as well as communal experience.
Clients may have already provided for their spiritual needs in a manner satisfactory to themselves.	The client's chosen way of meeting spiritual needs should be honored by nurses.
The spiritual needs of clients can vary throughout the course of an illness.	Nurses need to be alert to the varying spiritual concerns that may be expressed at different phases of an illness.
Spiritual needs can arise at any time on any day.	A caring environment should be in place to enhance and promote spiritual work at any time.
Humans have diverse beliefs, understandings, and levels of spiritual development.	Nurses should be encouraged to understand various belief systems and to understand a client's interpretation of them.
Clients and their families may have divergent spiritual beliefs, and they may not be aware of these differences.	Nurses should be aware of differences in spirituality within a family or close relationship and be alert to any difficulties that might ensue.

Box 1-5. Selected Assumptions and Principles of Spiritual Care *(concluded)*

The degree to which the client and family wish to examine and share spiritual matters is highly individual.	Nurses must be nonintrusive and sensitive to individual desires.
Clients are not always aware of, nor are able, nor wish to articulate spiritual issues.	Nurses should be aware and sensitive to unexpressed spiritual issues, and provide access to resources for clients who want to explore and communicate about spiritual issues.
Much healing and spiritual growth can occur in a client without assistance. Many people do not desire or need professional assistance in their spiritual development.	Acknowledgment and affirmation of a client's beliefs or spiritual concerns should be offered and may be all that is needed.

Source: Copyright 1990. Assumptions and principles of spiritual care. *Death Studies, 14*(1), 75–81. Reproduced by permission of Taylor & Francis, Inc., http://www.routledge-ny.com.

KEY POINTS

- Several nurse authors have proposed definitions for spirituality. Several nurse scholars have conducted analyses of the concept of spirituality. These definitions and analyses provide a clearer understanding of this broad, ethereal concept.
- Multiple concepts and terms related to spirituality are present in nursing literature. Clarification of these diverse terms will allow nurses to communicate more effectively with each other and with clients about their spiritual needs.

- Recent nursing literature is careful to distinguish religion from spirituality. It is also beginning to use broad, encompassing language to refer to that which is transcendent.
- Religion, culture, the psychosocial dimension, morality, and ethics are distinct from, yet related to, spirituality.
- There are innumerable ways in which spirituality may manifest clinically. Nursing diagnosis literature that presents "defining characteristics" and nursing research that has surveyed clinicians have identified similar manifestations of spiritual need.
- Spiritual development coincides with human development. Fowler's stages of faith development illustrate how people's spirituality develops.
- Nurses inevitably hold helpful and unhelpful assumptions about client spirituality and spiritual caregiving.

LOOK WITHIN TO LEARN

1. How do you define spirituality? Spiritual care? How will your definition of spirituality influence your attitudes about providing spiritual care?

2. With which of the assumptions about spiritual care for clients and family caregivers (listed in Box 1-5) do you agree? Why?

3. How does your culture and/or religion affect your spirituality? How might these religio-cultural factors influence the way you relate to clients from a different religio-cultural background?

4. Considering Fowler's stages of faith development, what stage best describes where you are spiritually? How might your stage of spiritual development affect your spiritual caregiving? How can you deliver spiritual care to a client who is at a different stage of spiritual development?

REFERENCES

Bold print indicates those that are most recommended.

Amenta, M. O. (1986). Spiritual concerns (Chapter 9, pp. 115–161). In M. O. Amenta & N. Bohnet (Eds.), *Nursing care of the terminally ill.* Boston: Little, Brown.

Burkhardt, M. A. (1989). Spirituality: An analysis of the concept. *Holistic Nursing Practice, 3*(3), 69–77.

Colliton, M. (1981). The spiritual dimension of nursing. In I. Beland & J. Y. Passos (Eds.), *Clinical Nursing* (4th ed.). New York: Macmillan.

Cushman, L., Wade, C., Factor-Litvak, P., Kronenberg, F., & Firester, L. (1999). Use of complementary and alternative medicine among African-American and Hispanic women in New York City: A pilot study. *Journal of the American Medical Women's Association, 54*, 193–195.

Didomizio, D. (1983). Sexuality. In G. Wakefield (Ed.), *A Dictionary of Christian Spirituality.* London: SCM Press.

Dombeck, M. B. (1996). Chaos and self-organization as a consequence of spiritual disequilibrium. *Clinical Nurse Specialist, 10*(2), 69–75.

Dossey, B. M., & Guzzetta, C. E. (2000). Holistic nursing practice (Chapter 1). In B. M. Dossey, L. Keegan, & C. E. Guzzetta (Eds.), *Holistic nursing: A handbook for practice* (3rd ed., pp. 5–26). Rockville, MD: Aspen.

Dyson, J., Cobb, M., & Forman, D. (1997). The meaning of spirituality: A literature review. *Journal of Advanced Nursing, 26*, 1183–1188.

Ellison, C. W. (1983). Spiritual well-being: Conceptualization and measurement. *Journal of Psychology & Theology,* 11, 330–340.

Emblen, J. D. (1992). Religion and spirituality defined according to current use in nursing literature. *Journal of Professional Nursing, 8*(1), 41–47.

Emblen, J. D., & Halstead, L. (1993). Spiritual needs and interventions: Comparing the views of patients, nurses, and chaplains. *Clinical Nurse Specialist, 7,* 175–182.

Fawcett, J., & Downs, F. S. (1992). *The relationship of theory and research* (2nd ed.). Philadelphia: Davis.

Ferrell, B. R., Grant, M., Funk, B., Garcia, N., Otis-Green, S., & Schaffner, M. L. J. (1996). Quality of life in breast cancer. *Cancer Practice, 4,* 331–340.

Fitchett, G., Burton, L. A., & Sivan, A. B. (1997). The religious needs and resources of psychiatric inpatients. *Journal of Nervous and Mental Diseases, 185,* 320–326.

Fowler, J. W. (1981). *Stages of faith development: The psychology of human development and the quest for meaning.* San Francisco: Harper & Row.

Fowler, M., & Peterson, B. S. (1997). Spiritual themes in clinical pastoral education. *Journal of Training and Supervision in Ministry, 18,* 46–54.

Goldberg, B. (1998). Connection: An exploration of spirituality in nursing care. *Journal of Advanced Nursing, 27,* 836–842.

Haase, J., Britt, T., Coward, D. D., Leidy, N. K., Penn, P. E. (1992). Simultaneous concept analysis of spiritual perspective, hope, acceptance, and self-transcendence. *Image: The Journal of Nursing Scholarship, 24,* 141–147.

Hermann, C. P. (2001). Spiritual needs of dying patients: A qualitative study. *Oncology Nursing Forum, 28,* 67–72.

Higgins, P. G., & Learn, C. D. (1999). Health practices of adult Hispanic women. *Journal of Advanced Nursing, 29,* 1105–1112.

Highfield, M. F., & Cason, C. (1983). Spiritual needs of patients: Are they recognized? *Cancer Nursing, 6,* 187–192.

Hood Morris, L. E. (1996). A spiritual well-being model: Use with older women who experience depression. *Issues in Mental Health Nursing, 17,* 439–455.

International Work Group on Death, Dying, and Bereavement. (1990). Assumptions and principles of spiritual care *Death Studies, 14,*(1), 75–81.

Jourard, S. (1964). *The transparent self: Self disclosure and well being.* New York: Van Nostrand, Reinhold.

Juarez, G., Ferrell, B., & Borneman, T. (1998). Influence of culture on cancer pain management in Hispanic patients. *Cancer Practice, 6,* 262–269.

Kim, M. J., McFarland, G. K., & McLane, A. M. (Eds.). (1991). Pocket guide to nursing diagnosis. (4th ed.). St. Louis, MO: Mosby.

Koenig, H., & Pritchett, J. (1998). Religion and psychotherapy. In H. Koenig (Ed.), *Handbook of religion and mental health* (Chapter 22). San Diego, CA: Academic Press.

Lee, M., Lin, S., Wrensch, M., Adler, S., & Eisenberg, D. (2000). Alternative therapies used by women with breast cancer in four ethnic populations. *Journal of the National Cancer Institute, 92*(1), 42–47.

Leininger, M. M. (1988). Leininger's theory of nursing: Cultural care diversity and universality. *Nursing Science Quarterly, 1,* 152–160.

Mansen, T. J. (1993). The spiritual dimension of individuals: Conceptual development. *Nursing Diagnosis, 4,* 140–147.

Martsolf, D. S. (1997). Cultural aspects of spirituality in cancer care. *Seminars in Oncology Nursing, 13,* 231–236.

Mayer, J. (1992). Wholly responsible for a part, or partly responsible for a whole? The concept of spiritual care in nursing. *Second Opinion, 17*(3), 26–55.

McMillan, S. C., & Weitzner, M. (2000). How problematic are various aspects of quality of life in patients with cancer at the end of life? *Oncology Nursing Forum, 27,* 817–823.

McSherry, W. (1998). Nurses' perceptions of spirituality and spiritual care. *Nursing Standard, 13*(4), 36–40.

McSherry, W., & Draper, P. (1998). The debates emerging from the literature surrounding the concept of spirituality as applied to nursing. *Journal of Advanced Nursing, 27,* 683–691.

Moadel, A., Morgan, C., Fatone, A., Grennan, J., Carter, J., Laruffa, G., Skummy, A., & Dutcher, J. (1999). Seeking meaning and hope: Self-reported spiritual and existential needs among an ethnically-diverse cancer patient population. *Psycho-Oncology, 8,* 378–385.

Narayanasamy, A. (1999). ASSET: A model for actioning spirituality and spiritual care education and training in nursing. *Nurse Education Today, 19,* 274–285.

Nolan, P., & Crawford, P. (1997). Towards a rhetoric of spirituality in mental health care. *Journal of Advanced Nursing, 26,* 289–294.

O'Brien, M. E. (1999). *Spirituality in nursing: Standing on holy ground.* Sudbury, MA: Jones and Bartlett.

Pargament, K. I. (1997). *The psychology of religion and coping.* New York: Guilford.

Potts, R. G. (1996). Spirituality and the experience of cancer in an African-American community: Implications for psychosocial oncology. *Journal of Psychosocial Oncology, 14*(1), 1–19.

Reed, P. G. (1992). An emerging paradigm for the investigation of spirituality in nursing. *Research in Nursing and Health, 15,* 349–357.

Smith, J. Z. (Ed.). (1995). The HarperCollins dictionary of religion. San Francisco: HarperSan Francisco.

Spilka, B., Spangler, J. D., & Nelson, C. B. (1983). Spiritual support in life threatening illness. *Journal of Religion and Health, 22(2),* 98–104.

Stallwood, J., & Stoll, R. (1975). Spiritual dimensions of nursing practice. In I. L. Beland & J. Y. Passos (Eds.), *Clinical nursing: Pathophysiological and psychosocial approaches* (pp. 1086–1098). New York: Macmillan.

Stoll, R. I. (1983). Emotional and spiritual support. In T. C. Kravis & C. G. Warner (Eds.), *Emergency medicine: A comprehensive review.* Rockville, MD: Aspen.

Stoll, R. I. (1989). The essence of spirituality. In V. B. Carson (Ed.), *Spiritual dimensions of nursing practice* (pp. 4–23). Philadelphia: Saunders.

Taylor, E. J., Highfield, M., & Amenta, M. (1994). Attitudes and beliefs regarding spiritual care: A survey of cancer nurses. *Cancer Nursing, 17*(6), 479–487.

Taylor, E. J., Amenta, M. O., & Highfield, M. F. (1995). Spiritual care practices of oncology nurses. *Oncology Nursing Forum, 22* **(1), 31–39.**

Vaillot, M. C. (1970). The spiritual factors in nursing. *Journal of Practical Nursing, 20,* 30–31.

Wan, G. J., Counte, M., Cella, D. F., Hernandez, L., McGuire, D. B., Deasay, S., Sshiomoto, G., & Hahn, E. (1999). The impact of socio-cultural and clinical factors on health-related quality of life reports among Hispanic and African-American cancer patients. *Journal of Outcome Measurement, 3,* 200–215.

2

Foundations for Spiritual Caregiving

Although there were times when the provision of spiritual care was not emphasized, spirituality has long been a part of nursing care. Recently, the relationship between spirituality and health has drawn considerable attention from researchers, health care practitioners, and consumers. By exploring historical, theoretical, and empirical bases for spiritual caregiving, this chapter provides a foundation on which to develop perspectives on the importance of spiritual caregiving.

In an effort to gain perspective, it is also helpful to examine current realities with regards to the provision of spiritual care. Nurses sometimes perceive barriers that prevent them from providing spiritual care (Taylor, Highfield, & Amenta, 1994; Sumner, 1998). They express this perception in statements like:

- "I don't know how to deal with someone's spirituality, and I don't feel comfortable doing it."
- "It's none of my business as a nurse."
- "Talking about religion or spirituality with clients is not appropriate."
- "It's more important to take care of the physiologic problems. There isn't enough time to take care of much else, never mind the spiritual problems."
- "You're not supposed to do it. That's what a boss told me once."

These statements suggest a fundamental question: Should nurses be involved in providing spiritual care to clients?

The purpose of this chapter is to present spiritual care as a core element of nursing care that deserves high priority. Historical, theoretical, professional, and empirical rationales support incorporating spiritual care in nursing practice. Likewise, there are reasons that underscore the need for health care institutions to provide spiritual care. Furthermore, many recipients of nursing care want to receive spiritual care.

HISTORICAL OVERVIEW OF SPIRITUALITY IN NURSING

When considering approaches to spiritual care that are appropriate and beneficial within the context of current times, a review of historical trends lends perspective. Nursing's earliest beginnings emerged within religious environments (Carson, 1989; Narayanasamy, 1999; O'Brien, 1999; Shelly & Miller, 1999). The essence of nursing is caring—nurturing others to promote well-being and providing support to those whose wellness is compromised. To do such work effectively, one must feel concern and compassion for others. For many nurses, this motivation to assist others arises from their spiritual core and reflects a need to give love.

Historically, family members, especially women, have provided nursing care. Presumably, nursing has existed whenever people were too sick or poor to care for themselves. Ancient records recount the provision of what would be described today as nursing care to individuals outside of an extended family. Lay attendants in Egyptian temples, priestesses in Babylonia, and people who assisted priest-physicians in early Palestinian, Chinese, and Indian civilizations functioned as nurses. The first biblical references to specific nurses include Rebekah's nurse (Genesis 24:59) and the Hebrew midwives Shiphrah and Puah (Exodus

1:15), whose clever reasoning before the Egyptian king saved the lives of Hebrew baby boys.

Some nurse historians assert that organized nursing began in response to Jesus Christ's teachings and role modeling (Shelly & Miller, 1999). Early Christians (e.g., deacons and deaconesses, Roman matrons), who organized themselves to provide aid to the poor and nurse the sick and disabled, believed that they were not only emulating the love of Jesus Christ, but also were serving God.

During the Middle Ages (around 500–1500 C.E.), those who chose to serve God through nursing entered monasteries (e.g., Benedict's or Francis of Assisi's) or military nursing orders (e.g., Knights Hospitallers of St. John of Jerusalem, Teutonic Knights), created to care for pilgrims to the Holy Land or those wounded in the Crusades. During this period, monastics founded hospitals (e.g., Hotel-Dieu in Paris, in 650 C.E.) for the indigent who were cared for by religious, humanitarian men and women. Many stories recount tales of devoted women who as nurses dedicated their wealth, influence, intellect, and energy to serving others. The motives and meaning of nursing during this period are expressed in the famous prayer attributed to St. Francis of Assisi (born 1184; see Box 2-1; Van de Weyer, 1993). This prayer undoubtedly inspired many monastic nurses of the Middle Ages, and it continues to be repeated by nurses and others today. (These words were sung at the funeral of Princess Diana, who like many noble women of the Middle Ages, devoted herself to helping marginalized people.)

During the Renaissance (1300–1600 C.E.) and post-Reformation eras (about 1500–1700 C.E.), the practice of nursing became increasingly institutionalized. In the 1500s, at least 100 religious orders were founded that essentially were communities of nurses (O'Brien, 1999). These nursing orders were both Protestant and Roman Catholic in orientation. One famous order founded in 1633 was the Daughters of Charity of St. Vincent de Paul. St. Vincent is credited with developing a model educational program. Criteria for becoming a Daughter of Charity included "good health, a sound mind, and a desire to serve God in a total way that involved teaching, nursing, and social service" (Narayanasamy, 1999, p. 391).

From the days of the Renaissance through the late 1800s, many who practiced nursing did so within a bleak environment. After the Reformation, many hospitals in Protestant areas formerly run by Roman Catholic monastics were closed or suppressed, which resulted in the deterioration of conditions and care. Difficult working conditions existed for nuns who worked in religious hospitals; they often were expected to work

Box 2-1. Prayer of St. Francis of Assisi

Lord, make me an instrument of your peace. Where there is hatred, let me sow love. Where there is injury, let me sow pardon. Where there is doubt, let me sow faith. Where there is despair, let me give hope. Where there is darkness, let me give light. Where there is sadness, let me give joy. O Divine Master, grant that I may Not try to be comforted, but to comfort; Not try to be understood, but to understand; Not try to be loved, but to love. Because it is in giving that we receive, in forgiving that we are forgiven, and in dying that we are born to eternal life.

Source: Van de Weyer, R. (1993). *The HarperCollins book of prayers: A treasury of prayers through the ages.* San Francisco: HarperSanFrancisco.

24-hour shifts and not touch any part of a client's body except the head and extremities (Shelly & Miller, 1999). More and more, nursing care was no longer associated with religious institutions; instead, nurses cared for people in homes and poorhouses. Nurses who did not belong to a religious order were often uneducated and sometimes corrupt. Dickens's infamous character, an uncaring, alcoholic nurse, Sairy Gamp, illustrated in *Martin Chuzzlewit* the wretched state of nursing during this period.

A primary proponent of health care reform, introduced during the nineteenth century in the United States and Europe, was Florence Nightingale (1820–1910). Nightingale received her nursing preparation from two religious institutions, the Kaiserwerth Institute for Deaconesses (Lutheran) and the Daughters of Charity of St. Vincent de Paul (Roman Catholic). Nightingale, a deeply spiritual and Christian woman and considered by some a mystic, helped to reform nursing by introducing the science of hygiene and by attracting and educating women considered moral and upstanding in their communities. Nightingale advocated holistic nursing, asserting that the spiritual dimension is an integral part of being human and spiritual care is essential to healing (O'Brien, 1999; Macrae, 1995).

For the first few decades of the twentieth century, nurses continued to openly acknowledge and follow religious precepts as part of their practice. Nursing literature of the early 1900s reveals tension between two ideas: nursing as a spiritual calling to service versus nursing as a profession that affords personal reward. Early articles of the *American Journal of Nursing* exemplify the tendency for nurse leaders to promote "ethical" nursing as Christian service. Box 2-2 provides several quotes that illustrate the influence of religious beliefs on attitudes about the "high calling" of nursing.

By the mid-twentieth century, religion became less visible as a component of nursing: The development of modern scientific methods and technological advances in health care served to devalue interventions that could not be easily controlled or quantified, including those essential to spiritual caregiving. Technological advances emphasized the "doing" rather than "being" aspects of nursing. The interest of government and nonsectarian entities in providing health care for a profit may also have contributed to the diminished influence of religion on nursing practice.

Over the last two decades, however, a renewed interest in the spirituality of nursing and the provision of spiritual care has emerged. Barnum (1996) asserted that this renewed focus on spirituality within nursing is explained by an increasing appreciation of nonrational phenomena, the spiritual emphasis of popular self-help programs, and the energetic advocacy of some within nursing (including traditionally religious nurses). This renewed focus on spirituality has been evidenced by increased numbers of presentations at professional nursing conferences about spiritual care, new courses or curricular themes about spirituality in nursing programs, and the formation of special interest groups devoted to spiritual care within professional organizations. Another indicator of nursing's renewed interest in spirituality has been the exponential growth in the number of nursing research reports on spirituality. The number of articles listed under the subject heading of "spirituality" by CINAHL (Cumulative Index to Nursing and Allied Health Literature) in 1982 was 14, in 1992 was 66, and in 1999 was 174. Editors of several major nursing journals have written editorials arguing the importance of spiritual care (e.g., Brink & Clark, 1994; Henry, 1995; Rothrock, 1994). In recent years, those who have written about spirituality in nursing have consistently agreed that to be effective, nursing care must include attention to nurse and client spirituality (e.g., O'Neill & Kenny, 1998; Wright, 1998).

Box 2-2. Associating Nursing with Christian Service: Excerpts from the *American Journal of Nursing* (1900–1910)

Volume 1, 1901, p. 104: Nursing "should be entrusted to women, each one of whom should be ordained a priestess, as it were, before she presumes to enter into the temple to perform her ministries unto sick and suffering humanity." [Final paragraph to a presidential address by Isabel H. Robb]

Volume 4, 1904, p. 520: "The great army of self sacrificing workers in this profession need no defense or public recognition. . . . Their reward is sufficient in knowing simply that they are helping those more needy than themselves. . . . If record is made, it is made by Him who said, 'Inasmuch as ye have done it unto one of the least of these, ye have done it unto Me.'" ["Ethics of Nursing" by Francis M. Quaife, superintendent of a training school in New Orleans]

Volume 5, 1905, p. 880: "We can each be faithful to duty . . . and when the Book of Life is unrolled, may we not hope to find our names there because 'Inasmuch as ye have done it unto one of the least. . . .' Our highest work as nurses is not simply to use technical skill we have acquired, but to so influence the lives of our patients as to inspire or aid them to a better and higher existence. The healing of the body may prove but the channel through which we may reach that which is infinitely greater—the spirit. We are dealing with great issues—those of life and death. . . ." ["Our Duty in Small Things" by Alice Luca, read at the Graduate Nurses Association]

Volume 6, 1906, p. 164–166: "In ethics, you cannot better the Golden Rule. . . . Does the thought of servitude depress you? Remember the ministering of Christ. Was not His whole life one of service? . . . pattern after no human model, but follow in the footsteps of Him who would 'heal the sick—and bind up the broken hearted'." [Address to the Colorado State Nurses Association entitled "Ethics in Private Practice" by Helen S. Thompson]

THEORETICAL FOUNDATIONS FOR SPIRITUAL CARE

Tracing nursing's history provides an understanding for how spirituality and religion have shaped nursing. Although nursing's historical tradition supports the inclusion of spiritual care as part of holistic nursing practice, tradition is a weak basis for determining practice. It is therefore important to review theoretical rationales that support the value of spiritual care.

Whole Person Care as the Essence of Nursing Care

Common to all nursing theories is the assumption that human beings comprise various dimensions and that each dimension is related to health and well-being. Many nursing theorists recognize clients as bio-psycho-social-spiritual beings, and while some have developed ways to categorize various human dimensions, all recognize multiple aspects of being human and advocate the provision of holistic care (Barnum, 1996; Dossey, Keegan, & Guzzetta, 2000).

To be considered holistic, nursing care must address health issues that arise from each human dimension and recognize the impact of one dimension on others. If a person's physiological well-being is challenged by the presence of a pathogen, psycho-social-spiritual dimensions of health will be affected. Someone who is experiencing the emotion of depression may feel physically sluggish and be searching for answers to relieve spiritual doubts or spiritual questions. Someone who has become disturbed by an uncomfortable sense of an inner void or ecstatic about a religious or spiritual experience will be affected across all dimensions.

Most people have experienced a connection between their spirits and how they feel physically or psychosocially. A nursing student who questions long-held religious or spiritual views after caring for a suffering child, for example, may feel tense or be unable to concentrate on other things. Or a nurse who is chronically fatigued may become irritable with her family and notice a lack of zest or enthusiasm for living.

Spiritual Component of Nursing

Several theoretical nursing models explicitly or implicitly identify spirituality as an aspect of nursing practice. These theories typically acknowledge spirituality when they discuss the nature of the nurse and nursing care, or when they describe the nature of the recipient of nursing care—the client. Because these are theories rather than concrete facts or practice protocols, they serve to establish a system of assumptions and principles and thus do not address practical specifics about spiritual caregiving. Theories do, however, provide a foundation for guidelines for spiritual caregiving that will be explored throughout this book. Selected nursing theories that speak to the importance of spiritual care are profiled here.

Henderson (1966) identified 14 specific activities that nurses should assist clients to carry out, one of which is to be able to worship according to one's faith. Henderson lists three other abilities that have a more tangential relation to spirituality, which are the ability to communicate to express feelings and thoughts, the ability to play and recreate, and the ability to learn and satisfy curiosity. Thus, spiritual care would entail assisting individuals to worship, pursue recreational activities, and so forth.

Travelbee (1971) defined nursing as "an interpersonal process whereby the professional nurse practitioner assists an individual, family, or community to prevent or cope with the experience of illness and suffering and, if necessary, to find meaning in these experiences" (p. 7). Travelbee recognizes that humans are motivated by meaning and that experiences that nurses witness and assist clients through (e.g., illness) are opportunities for creating meaning. Nursing care, Travelbee posits, should involve instilling hope. Furthermore, Travelbee asserts that a nurse can assist a client to find meaning only if the nurse "truly believes that meaning can be found" (p. 164). Although Travelbee does not use the word *spirituality,* the need to make sense of suffering, find meaning in life, and have hope are salient spiritual needs.

Watson's (1999) theory of human caring is another nursing theory frequently cited to support holistic practice, especially spiritual caregiving. Watson recognized that society needs, yet currently misses, the universal, mysterious, and powerful forces of love and care. Persons need to be cared for, loved, understood, accepted, and valued, to find harmony with life. The goal of nursing, according to Watson, is to help people achieve "a higher degree of harmony within the mind, body, and soul which generates self-knowledge, self-reverence, self-healing, and self-care processes" (p. 49). Nursing approaches that support this goal include allowing the client to express deep, inner feelings and communicating a feeling for and union with the client. Caring, as Watson describes it, is fundamentally a spiritual act that assists clients to achieve a greater sense of self as well as more harmony with body, mind, and soul. Watson believes that disharmony within a person's mind, body, and spirit, or between the person and the environment can lead to inner distress, illness, and possibly disease.

Neuman (1995) maintains that each person (or group of persons) constitutes a system of five variables: physiological, psychological, socio-

Box 2-3. Applying Nursing Theory to Practice

A 26-year-old woman is admitted to the surgical unit after having just had an appendectomy. The surgeon has ordered intravenous antibiotics and pain medication for surgical pain. A standard postoperative care plan is to be implemented to avoid atelectasis and other complications.

Travelbee

A nurse influenced by Travelbee's theory about nursing would make an effort to ascertain what the meaning of this experience was for the client. If the client were found to have an unanswered "why?" question, the nurse would provide assistance in a manner that exuded confidence that meaning could be created. The nurse would relate to the client as a fellow human, as a member of a symmetric dyadic relationship. Thus, in addition to using psychomotor skills to provide assistance with recovering from a medical intervention, the nurse would provide spiritual care primarily through the modality of verbal communication to assist the client to make sense of this life experience.

Neuman

A nurse who allows Neuman's Systems Model to guide practice would assess the level of spiritual awareness or development and address any identifiable spiritual needs occurring in reaction to the stress of surgery. The nurse would discuss with the client what spiritual resources and goals she possessed with the goal of achieving spiritual health. Activities that encourage increased spiritual awareness and meet client goals (e.g., reading, discussions with a spiritual mentor, meditation, clergy visitation) could be suggested.

Watson

A nurse guided by Watson's theory of Human Caring would give attention to personal spiritual development so as to be able to love and care for clients like this young woman. When delivering postoperative care, the nurse would, by her therapeutic presence, verbal and nonverbal communication, silence, or movement, connect with the client in a way that encourages her to express her deepest feelings.

cultural, developmental, and spiritual. These variables exist along a developmental continuum. The spiritual continuum can range from lack of awareness or denial of spirituality to a highly developed spiritual consciousness. To promote client wellness within an environment of stressors, the nurse must attend to all variables, including the spiritual. Fulton (1995) extends Neuman's theory by suggesting that providing spiritual care can strengthen client defenses against stressors.

All theories portray a unique picture that can guide nursing practice. Some nurses draw from more than one theory to develop effective approaches to client care. It is helpful to understand the assumptions behind the theory they select because these will determine the way they view themselves and provide care. The variation with which selected nursing theories can guide spiritual care is illustrated in Box 2-3.

Supportive Theories in Other Disciplines

Many theories developed outside of the discipline of nursing also provide support for spiritual care for those facing health challenges. Selected theories from the fields of sociology, psychiatry, and psychology share a theme, the human need for meaning, which fundamentally is a spiritual need. Thus, by discussing the need for persons to have meaning, these social scientists depict a salient aspect of spirituality and imply that it is a need with which people can be assisted.

Frankl (1985), the founder of logotherapy (a type of psychiatric therapy), maintained that the need for meaning was the primary motivating force in people's lives. Frankl suggested that people are able to find meaningfulness and can do so by (1) what they take from the world (e.g., enjoying the pleasures of nature or receiving the love of others), (2) what they give to the world (e.g., befriending and helping others), and (3) the attitude they choose for themselves in response to suffering. Frankl's thinking has influenced a number of nurse researchers who have explored how those with serious illness are able to attribute positive meanings to their illness (e.g., Taylor, 1993).

Sociologist Peter Marris (1986) studied numerous situations in which individuals experienced a significant loss or change (e.g., loss of a spouse, forced urban relocation from a rural setting). Marris identified that common to these varied circumstances was the need to recreate meaning after it had been challenged. Most health challenges that nurses address represent some type of client loss or change. Marris's theory guides the nurse to recognize the loss (e.g., death, diminished physical function, or loss of social contact) or change (e.g., change in lifestyle, comfort level, sleep pattern, or social roles) and help the client to reconstruct meaning within the client's new circumstances.

Similarly, psychologist Ronnie Janoff-Bulman (1992) theorized that all individuals hold a set of assumptions about the degree to which the world is beneficent and meaningful and their self-worth within it. A traumatic life event can shatter these assumptions. When this occurs, the individual will attempt to recreate meaning. A serious illness, for example, can alter assumptions that the world is a good place to be, life is meaningful, and one is a good person. Within the context of this theory, effective spiritual care would strive to help the client to recreate satisfactory assumptions after the crisis.

Lazarus's stress and coping framework (Lazarus & Folkman, 1984) is a psychological theory that has influenced some nurse researchers who have investigated spiritual responses to illness. This theory proposes that stress occurs when an event is evaluated as harmful or threatening (i.e., primary appraisal). During secondary appraisal, an individual assesses the availability and efficacy of resources for coping with the stressor. Coping strategies can include problem- or emotion-focused coping strategies. Following this framework, spiritual beliefs and practices can be viewed as coping strategies. For example, prayer might be used as a problem-focused coping strategy for physical healing or as an emotion-focused coping strategy for learning to live with an illness.

PROFESSIONAL MANDATES FOR SPIRITUAL CARE

The theoretical support for spiritual caregiving is recognized by professional organizations that influence nursing practice and education. Some professional organizations have issued mandates that direct nurses to offer spiritual care to clients and to teach spiritual care to students. The most influential of these is the JCAHO's mandate.

JCAHO Standards

The Joint Commission on Accreditation for Healthcare Organizations (JCAHO) specifies that all clients should be assessed for spiritual beliefs and practices and should have available spiritual support. Considering that the JCAHO is the accrediting body for all health care institutions wishing to receive reimbursements from Medicare, Medicaid, Social Security payments, and many third-party payers, this is a mandate that should motivate hospital administrators to support nurses and other health care professionals to attend to spiritual needs of clients carefully.

The JCAHO specifies that "spiritual assessments should, at a minimum, determine the patients denomination, beliefs, and what spiritual practices are important to the patient" (online, *http://www.jcaho.org/standard/ clarif/pe_spirtass.html*). The standards allow for each institution to determine exactly how and who will do these assessments. The JCAHO manual (2000) also stipulates in its section on "Patient Rights and Organization Ethics" that hospitals must demonstrate respect for clients' spiritual needs by providing "pastoral care and other spiritual services for patients who request them" (p. 80). The JCAHO also mandates that hospitals must respond to the spiritual concerns of dying clients and their families.

Nursing Mandates

Codes that guide the ethical conduct in nursing underscore the value nurses place on respecting all persons, regardless of their spirituality or religiosity. The American Nurses Association *Code for Nurses* (1985) states that nurses will respect the dignity and uniqueness of each client regardless of personal attributes. It is reasonable to infer from this statement that personal attributes include spiritual or religious preferences or affiliations. The International Council of Nurses *Code for Nurses* (2000) states that "the nurse promotes an environment in which the human rights, values, customs and spiritual beliefs of the individual, family and community are respected." The spirit of these mandates for nursing practice is echoed in directives that advise nursing educators to provide students with competency in physiologic, psychosocial, and spiritual care (Ross, 1996); that is, in the United States, the American Association of Colleges of Nursing, and in Great Britain, the United Kingdom Central Council for Nursing, Midwifery and Health Visiting.

EMPIRICAL SUPPORT FOR SPIRITUAL CARE

While nursing history and theory support the integration of spiritual care within nursing practice, an even stronger rationale is the mounting empirical evidence linking spirituality and health. Research suggests that spirituality and religiosity may protect a person from illness. Ample evidence demonstrates that people use spiritual and religious strategies for healing purposes. Of 1,004 polled Americans, 77 percent believed that "God sometimes intervenes to cure people who have a serious illness" (Kaplan, 1996).

Hundreds of studies have investigated relationships among spiritual, physical, and mental health variables (see Chapter 10). Those who have analyzed current research suggest that various indicators of spirituality and religiosity (an expression of spirituality) are often, but not always, associated with physical and mental health. That is, spiritual well-being is often positively correlated with physical and mental wellness. Religiosity is often associated with physical, social, and mental wellness. Some research (Fetzer Institute, 1999) suggests that there may be a predictive relationship between various aspects of religiosity or spirituality and:

- Enhanced subjective states of well-being
- Lower levels of depression and psychological distress
- Reduced mortality
- Delayed morbidity

Typically, research analyses include critiques of the research methods employed. As with many topics, spirituality, religiosity, and health present inherent difficulties for researchers. Research to investigate the relationships among these topics is especially challenging. Accusations about faulty assumptions or research methods employed can undermine results (e.g., Sloan, Bagiella, & Powell, 1999). Challenges that researchers must address include how to define and measure an aspect of spirituality, avoid introducing personal bias, and control confounding variables (Jarvis & Northcott, 1987; Sloan et al., 2000).

Increasingly, researchers from various disciplines are considering how to investigate the relationships between spirituality and health outcomes. One indication of this focus is an increase in the number of research instruments being developed to measure aspects of spirituality. To expand our knowledge about the impact of spirituality, we need to conduct nursing research that will investigate how aspects of spirituality influence responses to health challenges and identify the mechanisms that explain why spirituality influences health and how nursing interventions can promote spiritual health.

Spiritual Coping Strategies

Many researchers have asked study participants how they cope with health challenges. Whether the researcher asks open-ended questions or asks respondents to indicate the frequency with which they use various specified coping strategies, spiritual and religious coping strategies are usually identified (see Pargament, 1997, for a review). Sometimes, participants label the coping strategy simply as "faith." Other coping strategies that have a spiritual aspect include having hope and thinking positively. More specific spiritual coping strategies that researchers or participants identify are often religious in nature, such as reading religious materials and watching religious programs on television (e.g., Sodestrom & Martinson, 1987). Prayer is a frequently used coping strategy used by clients with various health concerns (see Chapter 9 for a complete review of this research).

Spirituality and Quality of Life

Nurses seek to assist clients to achieve quality of life, improve hardiness, attain psychosocial adjustment, and reduce anxiety and loneliness. Spiritual well-being and other aspects of spirituality appear to enhance these outcomes. Research demonstrates that spiritual variables are linked to other phenomena that determine quality of life. Examples of studies that support such linkages include the following, which suggest a positive correlation between a sense of spiritual well-being and:

- Quality of life, "fighting spirit," hope, and decreased negative mood states among persons experiencing cancer (e.g., Cotton, Levine, Fitzpatrick, Kold, & Targ, 1999; Fehring, Miller, & Shaw, 1997)
- Ability to predict "hardiness" in persons with aquired immune deficiency syndrome (AIDS) (Carson & Green, 1992)
- Reduced levels of uncertainty about illness among persons with diabetes mellitus (Landis, 1996)
- Reduced loneliness among chronically ill and healthy adults (Miller, 1985)
- Reduced anxiety among hospice patients (Kaczorowski, 1989)

Other variables related to spiritual well-being (e.g., sense of purpose in life, religiosity) have been positively correlated with psychosocial adjustment to illness (Mullen, Smith, & Hill, 1993; Taylor, 1993) and decreased perception of pain (Yates, Chalmer, St. James, Follansbee, & McKegney, 1981) among persons living with a cancer.

Economic Advantages

Advertisements (e.g., cars, shampoo) often suggest directly or indirectly that a product will enhance the buyer's sense of spiritual well-being.

Health care organizations are increasingly using this marketing tactic. In today's highly competitive health care market, health care systems, hospitals, and agencies vie for clients. One mark of quality some hospitals have touted is their intention to provide care for body, mind, and spirit.

An intervention found to reduce costs and improve client satisfaction and well-being would likely be embraced by most health care facilities. A scant amount of research indicates that supporting client spirituality can produce economic benefits. For example, in a study that illustrates how spiritual care can save money for a hospital, Florell (1973/1995) found evidence that daily chaplain visits can contribute to a decreased length of hospitalization, less anxiety related to surgery, lower consumption of pain medication, and fewer calls for nursing help. Other studies (e.g., Parkum, 1985) suggest that the presence of hospital chaplains contributes to client satisfaction and decreases the amount of litigation against the health care institution. It has also been observed that clients who receive pastoral care are more likely to return to the same hospital when they subsequently require care (VandeCreek, Jessen, Thomas, Gibbons, & Strasser 1991). Though dated, these studies are interesting and provide fertile ground for additional research.

Client Expectations with Regard to Spiritual Care

Another rationale for providing spiritual care is that many clients want spiritual care from their health care professionals. This presumably reflects the fact that most Americans consider themselves religious or spiritual. Polls consistently demonstrate that many Americans embrace religious and spiritual beliefs and practices. Gallup polls (1996) found at least 9 of every 10 American teens and adults believe in God (or a universal spirit), pray and believe their prayers have been answered, believe in a heaven, and state a religious preference. Other Gallup findings are presented in Box 2-4.

Clients generally report that they want health care professionals to tend to their spiritual needs. Two separate studies interviewed recipients of medical care in the southeastern United States and found that 73 percent and 77 percent of clients said that the physician should consider their spiritual needs or allow them to share their religious beliefs (Oyama & Koenig, 1998; King & Bushwick, 1994; respectively). Ehman and colleagues (1999) observed that 94 percent of 177 outpatient clinic clients indicated that they would welcome a carefully worded inquiry about their beliefs from their physician should they become gravely ill. Some studies have documented that clients frequently feel that not enough attention is

Box 2-4. Religiosity Among Adults in America

Basic Beliefs

83% believe that there is a God.

80% believe they have a personal relationship with God.

12% believe that there is a life force or spirit.

5% don't know or don't believe in a God or transcendent other.

65% believe in a devil.

90% believe in heaven.

73% believe in hell.

79% believe in miracles.

72% believe in angels.

27% believe in reincarnation.

23% believe in astrology.

80% expect to be called before God on Judgment Day.

61% believe the world will come to an end or be destroyed.

Religion

69% claim membership in a church, synogogue, or other religious body.

92% state a religious preference (58% are Protestant, 25% Roman Catholic, 2% are Jews, and less than 1% each state Hinduism, Buddhism, or Islam as a preference).

58% say religion is very important in their personal life (32% say it is fairly important).

61% say religion can answer all or most of today's problems.

57% have confidence in organized religion.

(continues)

paid their spiritual concerns (Anderson, Anderson, & Felsenthal, 1993; King & Bushwick). Two studies observed a direct relationship between client religiosity and client desire for a physician to discuss pertinent spiritual beliefs (Ehman et al.; Oyama & Koenig).

Box 2-4. Religiosity Among Adults in America *(continued)*

Worship Practices

31% say they usually attend church weekly.

75% pray at least daily.

95% say their prayers have been answered.

77% are satisfied with their prayer life.

37% wish their faith were stronger.

Source: Gallup, G. H., Jr. (1996). *Religion in America.* Princeton, NJ: Princeton Religion Research Center.

Several studies report that some clients use a form of "spiritual healing" to treat their diseases. For example, whereas 9 to 10 percent of a large sample from the general population saw a spiritual healer during the past year (Benson & Dusek, 1999; Eisenberg et al., 1993), 75 percent of osteoarthritis clients in another large sample reported that spiritual healers had been helpful (Rao et al., 1999). Astin (1998) identified several predictors that explain why Americans are increasingly utilizing complementary therapies such as spiritual healing and prayer. Predictive factors included having had an experience that altered the client's worldview and being interested in spirituality and personal growth.

An increasing number of nursing research studies describe client spiritual needs and show that hospitalization is a time when clients are vulnerable and receptive to spiritual care from a nurse (Bauer & Barron, 1995; Conco, 1995; Sodestrom & Martinson, 1987). Although it is thus far limited, evidence suggests that clients generally do not think of nurses as individuals from whom to receive spiritual nurture or guidance. When Bauer and Barron used a quantitative tool to survey 50 community-residing older adults about what spiritual care interventions they would prefer from a nurse, these researchers found that general attitudes of respect and caring were ranked higher than activities that were more overtly religious in nature. Top-ranked nursing activities included showing caring and respectful attitude, respecting religious beliefs, helping to promote hopefulness, listening when a client wants to talk, and treating religious articles and practices respectfully. Spiritual care interventions that received low rankings included encouraging exploration of spiritual issues, offering prayer, asking about relationship with or image of God or higher power, and helping to explore meaning in life.

Similar results were obtained in a study of 90 hospitalized adults completed in 1976 by Martin, Burrows, and Pomilio (in Fish & Shelly, 1978). When asked how they thought nurses could help to address spiritual needs, participants most frequently identified listening or allowing them to talk, calling clergy, and being kind and polite. Nearly every informant (97 percent) agreed that "nurses give spiritual care by being concerned, cheerful, and kind."

Furthermore, during three studies of persons living with cancer, nurse researchers obtained rankings for preferred spiritual care providers and found that nurses rank lower than family and friends and personal clergy but sometimes higher than chaplains and physicians (Highfield, 1992; Reed, 1991; Sodestrom & Martinson, 1987). These findings suggest that though many clients want and seek spiritual support, they may not always expect it from a nurse.

Conco (1995) observed that Christian clients value spiritual caregivers, regardless of their profession, who helped to:

- Enable transcendence to find greater meaning and purpose (e.g., by sharing personal experiences of making meaning when suffering)
- Enable hope (e.g., by sharing experiences of surmounting challenges)
- Establish connectedness (e.g., by being present, touching, accepting and understanding, self-disclosure, and sharing spiritual beliefs).

More than half of Sodestrom and Martinson's (1987) 25 informants agreed that it was important and appropriate for nurses to let clients talk about feelings toward God, and listen, make referrals to clergy, and allow privacy or assist clients with praying. Eleven of these 25 oncology patients also agreed that it was important and appropriate for nurses to acknowledge client religious beliefs and help clients with Bible reading if requested. Martin and colleagues (1976) results closely resemble Sodestrom and Martinson's and Conco's findings. That is, nursing interventions deemed as most appropriate by clients included listening (or allowing client to talk), calling clergy, and being "pleasant, kind, polite, and understanding." These data from different research studies, collected during three different decades, vary little.

IMPLICATIONS FOR NURSING PRACTICE

The need to incorporate spiritual care is grounded in nursing history and theory and reinforced by research and professional mandates. The implications for nursing practice that follow are drawn from these foundations.

The history of spiritual care in nursing should encourage nurses to examine and value the spiritual beliefs that motivate their work—or service—as nurses. History also suggests that organized religion may have a beneficial influence on creating an environment that fosters quality care and outreach to underserved populations. Religious health care centers and universities often provide supportive environments in which nurses may develop and teach best practices, particularly in the area of spiritual care.

A number of nurse theorists support the view that the spiritual dimension is an important component of holistic nursing care. Some propose that the nurse's spirituality contributes to the client's healing environment. Theories from social sciences posit that certain life events may challenge a client's spiritual beliefs and meanings. Effective nursing care requires that nurses prepare themselves to address client spiritual concerns. Clients may especially benefit from spiritual care when critical life events challenge assumptions about the world. As holistic nursing theory posits, spiritual needs do not occur in isolation. Health-related challenges often incorporate spiritual elements, and effective nursing care will address them. Loneliness that keeps a client awake at night, for example, may reflect a sense of neglect or betrayal of loved ones or the absence of God. A client in pain may also be struggling with questions such as "Why me?"

Research supports spiritual well-being as an important contributor to quality of life as well as the widespread use of spiritual resources to cope with life's challenges. Thus, nurses should strive to promote spiritual well-being and assist clients with coping strategies. Nurses should also support clergy, chaplains, and other experts in spiritual care who may provide invaluable support to clients. Because spiritual needs can emerge at any time and may sometimes require an immediate response, a nurse should be able to provide at least some basic level of spiritual care when a spiritual care expert is not immediately available.

Some research suggests that spiritual care (particularly that given by chaplains) may provide economic benefits to health care institutions. To increase the likelihood of client satisfaction with health care services and financial savings, nurses can collaborate with experts to provide spiritual care. Because spiritual care flourishes in an environment of rapport and trust and brief visits by spiritual care experts may not provide adequate time to build a relationship, it is important for nurses to be involved in spiritual caregiving. Clergy and chaplains typically carry very large caseloads and may serve hundreds of parishioners or hospitals with hundreds of beds. Spiritual care experts may find it difficult to make lengthy or frequent client visits.

Working at the bedside, however, the nurse can establish rapport and form a relationship with the client on which to continue spiritual care.

As the growing body of research indicates, many clients want their health care professionals to provide some attention to spiritual matters. Identifying and addressing spiritual needs is a fundamental part of nursing spiritual assessment (see Chapter 5). If clients do not always look to nurses when spiritual needs arise, evidence suggests that they value aspects of nursing care that are essentially spiritual care.

Because self-identified religious persons are more likely to value an overt discussion of health-related spiritual issues, nurses can generally approach spiritual care with religious clients more overtly. The religious client will likely be receptive to a spiritual assessment or the nurse's offer to share prayer or read a comforting passage from a holy book. Nonreligious clients are likely to respond better to nonreligious language. To promote effective communication regardless of client spiritual or religious orientation, in subsequent dialogue, the nurse strives to use language that incorporates client descriptions of spiritual concepts (see Chapter 4). Nonreligious clients may be more receptive to discussing spiritual concerns and coping strategies if the nurse prefaces the discussion with statements like:

- "Nurses recognize that there is a strong connection between how we feel physically, emotionally, and spiritually. Because how you're feeling spiritually can also influence how we care for you, it would help me to know of any spiritual concerns you may be wondering about."
- "Research tells us that many people draw on their spirituality to help them cope during times of difficulty. Are there spiritual practices that you might find comforting? How may I help you use them?"

Research indicates that clients perceive spiritual care to be beneficial, and there is no evidence of negative client perceptions of spiritual care received from nurses. Thus, a deficit in spiritual care may arise not from how nurses provide spiritual care but from the perception they do not care about a client's spiritual needs. Clients who perceive that nurses are too busy or unable to provide spiritual care may withhold spiritual concerns. Nurses can challenge this perception individually and collectively by consistently providing spiritual care and encouraging other nurses to do so.

Many clients view family, friends, and clergy as the most important spiritual care providers. Conco's (1995) informants identified nonprofessional hospital personnel as people who provided spiritual care. Nurses often recognize and research participants verify that housekeepers, transport workers, and other staff do provide emotional and spiritual support for hospitalized clients and their families. Nurses can play a vital role in guiding family and friends to offer spiritual care and in collaborating with clergy. Chapter 8 explores methods to support collaborative efforts.

Research indicates that clients sometimes do not want to discuss spirituality and do not rank their health care providers as primary spiritual care providers. It is important to recognize that some people do not feel comfortable talking about spirituality and that it is natural to consider family and clergy as primary spiritual care providers. These research findings may also reflect stereotypical perceptions that nurses and medical professionals are interested only in addressing physiologic problems and that disease is primarily a pathophysiologic phenomenon. By educating clients to appreciate the multidimensionality of health (e.g., its social, economic, cultural, and spiritual dimensions), nurses can encourage clients to perceive them as resources for spiritual care.

Nursing implications drawn from research on client expectations are summarized in Box 2-5.

Box 2-5. Nursing Implications Drawn from Research on Client Expectations

Research Finding	Nursing Implication
Many clients desire spiritual care from their health care professionals (e.g., open discussion of beliefs, prayer).	Nursing assessments should include questions about how clients want spiritual care from their nurses.
Religious clients are more likely to desire spiritual care from health care professionals.	Direct talk about spirituality will likely be welcomed more by religious clients. However, the nurse can discuss spiritual health matters with nonreligious clients after assessing how they describe spiritual concepts and using their terminology.

Box 2-5. Nursing Implications Drawn from Research on Client Expectations *(continued)*

For spiritual care, clients rank family, friends, and personal clergy higher than nurses and other health care professionals.	Nurses must support clients' family, friends, and clergy as primary spiritual care providers.
Clients value spiritual nursing care.	Nurses can earn clients' respect as spiritual care providers by providing excellent care and educating clients regarding the nurse's role in nurturing spiritual health.
Clients identify kind and respectful care as part of spiritual care.	Nurses should strive to provide "simple" kindnesses that demonstrate caring and boost client spirits.

KEY POINTS

- History, theory, and research offer rationale for including spiritual care in nursing practice.
- Nurses sometimes perceive barriers to providing spiritual care. These barriers include a perceived lack of time, ability, lack of knowledge and preparation for spiritual caregiving, orientation to nursing care that emphasizes the biologic, and confusion about what spiritual care is.
- The history of nursing is intertwined with religious history, particularly Christianity. A resurgence of interest in spirituality has emerged over the past decade.
- Rationales for nurses to provide spiritual care include:
  - An emphasis on holistic nursing care supported by nursing theory
  - Mandates from professional organizations dedicated to improving nursing practice and education

- Empirical research providing evidence that spirituality and religiosity are positively related to improved health outcomes and that clients value and frequently use spiritual coping strategies

- Evidence indicates that many clients want their health care practitioners to address spiritual concerns and also that not all clients do want this. Furthermore, clients often do not think of nurses as providers of spiritual care.

- Implications for nursing care drawn from history, theory, and research include:

  - The approach to spiritual caregiving should vary for religious and nonreligious clients.

  - Nurses can encourage client receptivity to spiritual care by educating clients about the multidimensionality of health.

  - Spiritual care should include supporting friends and family, as well as clergy and other spiritual care experts, as they care for a client.

- Their accessibility to clients affords nurses the opportunity to establish rapport that supports spiritual care.

LOOK WITHIN TO LEARN

1. In earlier times, many were motivated to become nurses by a calling to service. What motivated you to choose nursing? Do you view nursing as professional work, a calling to service, or in some other way?

2. How does the theoretical framework that guides your study and/or practice of nursing address the spiritual dimension and spiritual care? How does this framework influence spiritual caregiving that you provide?

3. If you were required to identify either the client's physical or spiritual dimension as the most important dimension for which to provide care, which would you choose? Why?

4. Some clients do not look to nurses to address their spiritual concerns. What can you do to encourage clients, including those who do not view themselves as religious, to be receptive to spiritual care from a nurse?

REFERENCES

Bold print indicates those that are most recommended.

American Nurses Association. (1985). *Code for nurses*. Kansas City, MO: American Nurses Publishing.

Anderson, J. M., Anderson, L. J., & Felsenthal, G. (1993). Pastoral needs and support within an inpatient rehabilitation unit. *Archives of Physical Medicine and Rehabilitation, 74,* 214–217.

Astin, J. A. (1998). Why patients use alternative medicine: Results of a national study. *Journal of the American Medical Association, 279,* 1548–1553.

Barnum, B. S. (1996). *Spirituality in nursing: From traditional to new age.* New York: Springer.

Bauer, T., & Barron, C. R. (1995). Nursing interventions for spiritual care: Preferences of the community-based elderly. *Journal of Holistic Nursing, 13,* 268–279.

Benson, H., & Dusek, J. A. (1999). Self-reported health, and illness and use of conventional and unconventional medicine and mind/body healing by Christian Scientists and others. *Journal of Nervous and Mental Disease, 187,* 539–548.

Brink, P. J., & Clark, M. B. (1994). Research in pastoral care. *Western Journal of Nursing Research, 16,* 129–131.

Carson, V. B. (Ed.) (1989). *Spiritual dimensions of nursing practice*. Philadelphia: Saunders.

Carson, V. B., & Green, H. (1992). Spiritual well-being: A predictor of hardiness in patients with acquired immunodeficiency syndrome. *Journal of Professional Nursing, 8,* 209–220.

Conco, D. (1995). Christian patients' views of spiritual care. *Western Journal of Nursing Research, 17,* 266–276.

Cotton, S. P., Levine, E. G., Fitzpatrick, C. M., Kold, K. H., & Targ, E. (1999). Exploring the relationships among spiritual well-being, quality of life, and psychological adjustment in women with breast cancer. *Psycho-Oncology, 8,* 429–438.

Dossey, B. M., Keegan, K., & Guzzetta C. E. (Eds.). (2000). *Holistic nursing: A handbook for practice* **(3rd ed.). Rockville, MD: Aspen.**

Ehman, J. W., Ott, B. B., Short, T. H., Ciampa, R. C., & Hansen-Flaschen, J. (1999). Do patients want physicians to inquire about their spiritual or religious beliefs if they become gravely ill? *Archives of Internal Medicine, 159,* 1803–1806.

Eisenberg, D. M., Kessler, R. C., Foster C., Norlock, F. E., Calkins, D. R., & Delbanco, T. L. (1993). Unconventional medicine in the United States: Prevalence, costs, and patterns of use. *New England Journal of Medicine, 328,* 246–252.

Fehring, R., Miller, J., & Shaw, C. (1997). Spiritual well being, religiosity, hope, depression and other mood states in elderly people coping with cancer. *Oncology Nursing Forum, 24,* 663–671.

Fetzer Institute. (1999). *Multidimensional measurement of religiousness/spirituality for use in health research: A report of the Fetzer Institute/National Institute on Aging Working Group.* **Author. [Available: 9292 West KL Avenue, Kalamazoo, MI 49009–9398].**

Fish, S., & Shelly, J. A. (1978). *Spiritual care: The nurse's role.* Downers Grove, IL: InterVarsity Press.

Florell, J. L. (1973/1995). Crisis intervention in orthopedic surgery: Empirical evidence of the effectiveness of a chaplain working with surgery patients. Reprinted from Bulletin of the American Protestant Hospital Association in L. VandeCreek (Ed.), *Spiritual needs and pastoral services: Readings in research* (Chapter 2, pp. 23–32). Decatur, GA: Journal of Pastoral Care Publications.

Frankl, V. (1985). *Man's search for meaning.* New York: Washington Square Press.

Fulton, R. B. (1995). The spiritual variable: Essential to the client system. In B. Neuman (Ed.), *The Neuman Systems Model (3rd ed.)*(pp. 77–91). Stamford, CT: Appleton & Lange.

Gallup, G. H., Jr. (1996). *Religion in America.* Princeton, NJ: Princeton Religion Research Center.

Henderson, V. A. (1966). *The nature of nursing: A definition and its implications for practice, research, and education.* Riverside, NJ: Macmillan.

Henry, B. (1995). The spiritual in nursing. *Image: The Journal of Nursing Scholarship, 27,* 86.

Highfield, M. F. (1992). Spiritual health of oncology patients: Nurse and patient perspectives. *Cancer Nursing, 15,* 1–8.

International Council of Nurses. (2000). *The ICN Code of Ethics for Nurses.* Available: http.//www.icn.ch/icncode.pdf

Janoff-Bulman, R. (1992). *Shattered assumptions: Towards a new psychology of trauma.* **New York: Free Press.**

Jarvis, G. K., & Northcott, H. C. (1987). Religion and differences in morbidity and mortalitiy. *Social Science and Medicine, 25,* 813–824.

Joint Commission on Accreditation for Health Care Organizations. (2000). *Hospital accreditation standards.* Oakbrook, IL: Author.

Kaczorowski, J. M. (1989). Spiritual well-being and anxiety in adults diagnosed with cancer. *Hospice Journal, 5,* 105–116.

Kaplan, M. (1996, June 24). Ambushed by spirituality. *Time, 148,* 62.

King, D. E., & Bushwick, B. (1994). Beliefs and attitudes of hospital inpatients about faith healing and prayer. *Journal of Family Practice, 39,* 349–352.

Landis, B. J. (1996). Uncertainty, spiritual well-being, and psychosocial adjustment to chronic illness. *Issues in Mental Health Nursing, 17,* 217–231.

Lazarus, R., & Folkman, S. (1984). *Stress, appraisal, and coping.* New York: Springer.

Marris, P. (1986). *Loss and change.* London: Routledge & Kegan Paul.

Martin, C., Burrow, C., & Pomilio, J. (1976). Spiritual needs of patients study (Appendix A, pp. 150–166). In S. Fish & J. A. Shelly (Eds.), *Spiritual care: The nurse's role.* Downers Grove, IL: InterVarsity Press.

Macrae, J. (1995). **Nightingale's spiritual philosophy and its significance for modern nursing.** *Image: Journal of Nursing Scholarship, 27,* 8–10.

Miller, J. F. (1985). Assessment of loneliness and spiritual well-being in chronically ill and healthy adults. *Journal of Professional Nursing, 1,* 79–85.

Mullen, P., Smith, R., & Hill, E. (1993). Sense of coherence as a mediator of stress for cancer patients and spouses. *Journal of Psychosocial Oncology, 11*(3), 23–46.

Narayanasamy, A. (1999). Learning spiritual dimensions of care from a historical perspective. *Nurse Education Today, 19,* 386–395.

Neuman, B. (1995). *The Neuman Systems Model* (3rd ed.). Stamford, CT: Appleton & Lange.

O'Brien, M. E. (1999). *Spirituality in nursing: Standing on holy ground.* Sudbury, MA: Jones and Bartlett.

O'Neill, D. P., & Kenny, E. K. (1998). Spirituality and chronic illness. *Image: The Journal of Nursing Scholarship, 30,* 275–280.

Oyama, O., & Koenig, H. G. (1998). Religious beliefs and practices in family medicine. *Archives of Family Medicine, 7,* 431–435.

Pargament, K. I. (1997). *The psychology of religion and coping.* New York: Guilford.

Parkum, K. H. (1985). The impact of chaplaincy services in selected hospitals in the Eastern United States. *Journal of Pastoral Care, 39,* 262–269.

Rao, J. K., Mihaliak, K., Kroenke, K., Bradley, J., Tierney, W. M., & Weinberger, M. (1999). Use of complementary therapies for arthritis among patients of rheumatologists. *Annuls of Internal Medicine, 131,* 409–416.

Reed, P. G. (1991). Preferences for spiritually related nursing interventions among terminally ill and nonterminally ill hospitalized adults and well adults. *Applied Nursing Research, 4,* 122–128.

Ross, L. A. (1996). Teaching spiritual care to nurses. *Nurse Education Today, 16,* 38–43.

Rothrock, J. C. (1994). The meaning of spirituality to perioperative nurses and their patients. *AORN Journal, 60,* 894–896.

Shelly, J. A., & Miller, A. B. (1999). *Called to care: A Christian theology of nursing.* Downers Grove, IL: InterVarsity Press.

Sloan, R. P., Bagiella, E., & Powell, T. (1999). Religion, spirituality, and medicine. *Lancet, 353,* 664–667.

Sloan, R. P., Bagiella, E., VandeCreek, L., Hover, M., Casalone, C., Hirsch, T. J., Hasan, Y., Kreger, R., & Poulos, P. (2000). Should physicians prescribe religious activities? *New England Journal of Medicine, 342,* 1913–1916.

Sodestrom, K. E., & Martinson, I. M. (1987). Patients' spiritual coping strategies: A study of nurse and patient perspectives. *Oncology Nursing Forum, 14,* 41–45.

Sumner, C. H. (1998). Recognizing and responding to spiritual distress. *American Journal of Nursing, 98,* 26–30.

Taylor, E. J. (1993). Factors associated with the sense of meaning among people with recurrent cancer. *Oncology Nursing Forum, 20*(9), 1399–1407.

Taylor, E. J., Highfield, M., & Amenta, M. (1994). Attitudes and beliefs regarding spiritual care: A survey of cancer nurses. *Cancer Nursing, 17*(6), 479–487.

Travelbee, J. (1971). Interpersonal aspects of nursing (2nd ed.). Philadelphia: Davis.

VandeCreek, L., Jessen, A., Thomas, J., Gibbons, J., & Strasser, S. (1991). Patient and family perceptions of hospital chaplains. *Hospital and Health Services Administration, 36,* 455–467.

Van de Weyer, R. (1993). The HarperCollins book of prayers: A treasury of prayers through the ages. San Francisco: HarperSanFrancisco.

Watson, J. (1999). *Nursing human science and human care: A theory of nursing.* Sudbury, MA: Jones and Bartlett.

Wright, K. B. (1998). **Professional, ethical, and legal implications for spiritual care in nursing.** *Image: Journal of Nursing Scholarship, 30,* 81–83.

Yates, J. W., Chalmer, B. J., St. James, P., Follansbee, M., & McKegney, F. P. (1981). Religion in patients with advanced cancer. *Medical and Pediatric Oncology, 9,* 121–128.

3

Spiritual Self-Awareness and Client Care

Developing spiritual self-awareness is an essential part of learning how to provide spiritual care to nursing clients. "To meet the spiritual needs of patients, nurses need to be aware of their own spirituality, either within a recognized religious framework or in less structured ways" (Danvers, 1998, p. 35). Some nurses may not think much about their own spirituality, or they may be uncomfortable with exploring their own spiritual thoughts, feelings, and beliefs. The nurse's awareness of his or her sense of the spiritual, however, has a profound influence on the ability to provide effective spiritual care.

Consider these illustrative scenarios:

- After openly discussing his sense of isolation from God with a spiritual mentor, a nurse discovers he is willing to listen to the spiritual pain of a client who volunteers, "Sometimes I wonder if God is with me."
- A nurse whose feelings were hurt by members of her church now believes that institutionalized forms of worship do not promote spiritual growth and avoids making referrals to chaplains and clergy for her patients, believing that she is acting in their best interest.

These examples show how the nurse's spiritual or religious beliefs can affect client care. Because spiritual self-awareness is essential to the provision of effective and ethical spiritual care, the purpose of this chapter is to explore how nurses can increase their level of spiritual self-awareness. After a review of theory and research that supports the importance of spiritual awareness among nurses, this chapter explores practical aspects of developing self-awareness as well as how nurses share their beliefs with clients. Sharing spiritual beliefs in an ethical manner can be beneficial to clients. It is also possible, however, for nurses to inappropriately impose their beliefs and practices on clients—an inappropriate approach to spiritual nursing care. This ethical issue of spiritual caregiving will be explored in depth.

SPIRITUAL SELF-AWARENESS: THEORY, RESEARCH, AND PRACTICE

Theory

Many nurse scholars (e.g., Danvers, 1998; Dossey, Keegan, & Guzzetta, 2000; Nagai-Jacobson & Burkhardt, 1989) posit that nurses must gain a degree of awareness about their own spirituality to be effective as spiritual caregivers. Several have adopted the metaphor "wounded healer" created by theologian Henri Nouwen (1979) to describe the nature of the nurse as a caregiver. A wounded healer is, like the client, wounded in some way—hurt, distressed, broken, scarred, or dis-eased. What allows wounded individuals to be effective as healers is the recognition of their own woundedness. Thus, the ability to embrace one's woundedness enhances the ability to heal.

"But I'm not wounded! I haven't had anything really bad happen to me," some may object. The wounded healer metaphor, however, applies to anyone who wants to care for and assist in the healing of others. Everyone experiences some degree of pain, whether the breakup of a romantic relationship, an unkind remark from a parent or friend, the loss of someone or something, or the experience of any unexpected or difficult transition. Even though a nurse may not have been diagnosed with physical or mental disease, he or she can on some level identify with the client's experience (e.g., a sense that the body betrayed him or her or feelings of loss and change). Recognition of shared woundedness encourages the nurse to be genuine, sensitive, and empathic.

Brittain (1986) maintained that "spiritual care is delivered as much by who one is as by what one says" (p. 115). Brittain's idea is supported by others who believe that spiritual care involves not only *doing* but also *being* (e.g., Dossey, Keegan, & Guzzetta, 2000; Mayer, 1992). Not only can nurses assist clients within a healing environment, but when they are able to be fully present, to intentionally focus and be receptive, their very presence actually contributes to the healing process. Thus, the therapeutic presence of the nurse serves as an instrument of healing (McKivergin, 2000; Quinn, 2000).

Quinn (2000) identified ways of being with clients that are unique to nurses who are able, with their presence, to create a healing environment. These ways of being or "holding sacred space" differ from a "getting the job done" attitude. For example, instead of leading and "doing for" the client, the nurse healer will walk beside and be with a client. Quinn believes that nurses who intentionally place themselves in a centered or meditative state can create an interconnectedness between the energy fields of both the nurse and the client. By doing this, the nurse can promote the client's ability to relax, rest, and heal. Questions that help a nurse to consider how well he or she is promoting a healing environment are presented in Box 3-1.

To be someone who by "simply" being present becomes an instrument for healing, it is essential to cultivate self-awareness. McKivergin (2000) identified characteristics that influence the nurse's ability to be an instrument of healing, including:

- Appreciation of self-healing as a constant process
- Openness to self-discovery
- Clearness about life's purposes in order to avoid perfunctory behavior and boredom

Box 3-1. Questions for Self-Assessment of Nurse Healers

- Do patients hear in my voice that I care? That I have time for them? That they are safe with me?
- What is the quality of my facial expression? Of my eyes? Do they communicate care and compassion, or are they perfunctory and distant? Does the patient feel seen by me, or overlooked? If the eyes are the windows of the soul, what is my soul saying to the soul of my patient? What is the patient's soul saying?
- Am I focused on the task at hand and simply touching the patient to get the job done? Or does my touch convey care, support, nurture, and competence? Does my touch communicate that I know I am touching this person's spirit as I contact his or her skin, because where else is the spirit located but in the body? Do I speak of love and kindness and respect through my hands? (pp. 45–46)

Source: Reprinted/adapted with permission from Dossey, *Holistic Nursing: A Handbook for Practice,* 3rd ed., pp. 45–46. ©2000, Aspen Publishers, Inc.

- Awareness of potential areas for personal growth so that insight about inner processes can be gained and shared
- Nurturing self so as to model self-care for clients
- Perceiving time with clients as an opportunity to serve and share with them

Theory that has emerged in nursing on the significance of self-awareness is supported by theologian Paul Dominic (1988). He suggested that in many faith traditions of the world, self-awareness is considered to be the most important contributor to spiritual growth. Self-awareness is essential to personal spirituality because, as he quotes a wise saying, "Unawareness is the root of all evil" (p. 749). Self-awareness involves bringing to focus what is really wanted, what is repulsive, what are one's biases and "hot buttons," what is thought, what is felt, and so forth. It is through this process of self-discovery that we learn the truth about who we are—that we become self-aware. Furthermore, for those who believe that God is imminent (exists within us rather than only externally), self-awareness reveals Self-awareness. That is, listening to what is within, to that "still small voice," Inner Wisdom, or Inward Light, may be a way to listen to and be aware of God.

Empirical Research

Much of the nursing literature that emphasizes the importance of spiritual self-awareness is "theoretical," based on the personal and experiential knowledge of expert nurses. Several nursing research studies validate the impact of nurses' spirituality on their nursing care. Soeken and Carson's (1986) study of nursing students demonstrated a positive correlation between self-reported spiritual well-being and attitudes toward spiritual caregiving. A few studies have documented a positive relationship between attitudes toward spiritual caregiving and actual delivery of spiritual care (Millison & Dudley, 1992; e.g., Piles, 1990; Taylor, Highfield, & Amenta, 1994). Some researchers have found that the degree of nurses' self-reported spirituality and religiousness is directly associated with the likelihood of assessing spiritual needs (Ross, 1994) and providing spiritual care (Taylor, Highfield, & Amenta, 1999). Before the Joint Commission on Accreditation for Healthcare Organizations (JCAHO) mandated spiritual assessment, Boutell and Bozett (1987) studied nurses who lived in the "Bible Belt" and observed that these predominantly religious nurses (74 percent were active in their religion) reported uncharacteristically high rates of spiritual assessment (i.e., 72 percent reported they did so at least occasionally). Taylor and colleagues' (1999) study is especially convincing (see Box 3-2); they observed that the degree to which nurses defined themselves as spiritual predicted their beliefs about spiritual care and their self-reported comfort and ability to give such care.

Research findings reveal that nurses often perceive they receive a positive spiritual benefit from caring for clients. Millison and Dudley (1990), for example, found from a survey of 120 hospice professionals (85 of whom were nurses) that 69 percent of respondents indicated that their work often had a positive effect on their personal spirituality. Likewise, Highfield, Taylor, & Amenta (2000) found that 65 percent of 813 oncology and hospice nurses reported that their patients had influenced their spirituality "a great deal." These nurses expressed that they learned from and were inspired by working with patients. Analysis of the narrative data from this study indicated how this positive influence emerged. Caring for cancer patients helped these nurses to:

- Examine and question their own beliefs
- Strengthen their beliefs
- Confront their own mortality and vulnerability
- Experience an increased appreciation for life and for people
- Cherish and live in the present

Box 3-2. Profile of Research: Predictors of Oncology and Hospice Nurses' Spiritual Care Perspectives and Practices

Purpose: To identify variables that predict nurses' attitudes about spiritual care and their spiritual care practices.

Method: Mailed surveys were completed by 181 oncology nurses and 638 hospice nurses. Surveys posed quantitative and open-ended questions assessing attitudes about, perceived frequency of, ability to, and comfort with spiritual caregiving. Demographic questions included five-point Likert scales to assess degree of personal spirituality and religiosity. Data analyses techniques included Pearson correlations and stepwise multiple regression.

Main Findings: Attitudes about spiritual caregiving were positively correlated with the self-reported frequency, ability, and comfort with which these nurses provided spiritual care (these correlations being between 0.43 and 0.50). Degree of personal spirituality explained the variation in nurses' attitudes more than any other variable. Attitudes about spiritual caregiving accounted for 25% of the variation in how frequently nurses provided spiritual care. Similarly, personal spirituality and perspectives about spiritual caregiving predicted most the self-reported ability and comfort with providing spiritual care.

Practice Application: Because nurses' degree of personal spirituality and their attitudes predict their spiritual caregiving practices, nurses must seriously consider how they can promote their own spiritual health and acquire positive perspectives about spiritual caregiving.

Source: Taylor, E. J., Highfield, M. F., & Amenta, M. O. (1999). Predictors of oncology and hospice nurses' spiritual care perspectives and practices. *Applied Nursing Research, 12,*(1), 30–37.

Guidelines for Promoting Self-Awareness

As indicated by theory and research, self-awareness is essential to spiritual experience and growth, and in turn, to providing effective spiritual care. Because spiritual care requires being present therapeutically, being aware of personal woundedness, and being spiritually sensitive, it follows that to be effective, nurses need to develop self-awareness. But how does one develop self-awareness? Several authors provide suggestions.

Watson (1999), a hospice counselor, agrees that nurses must become self-aware to care for others and advocates that nurses identify and address their feelings. Feelings, although they can sometimes distort, have a purpose. Feelings of grief help us to deal with our losses. Feelings of anger inform us of an injustice and energize us to take action to correct it. Recognizing our jealousy helps us learn that we want something. Fear helps us to be cautious. Feeling loved helps us to love others. To manage such feelings in ways that are healthy, Watson suggests that it is important to find "safe" persons and situations with whom to talk about these feelings. Telling one's story helps one to deal with and learn from feelings.

Spirituality is not separate from daily life. Several health care professionals remind us that a nurse can use ways of finding spirit at work or in daily life (e.g., having a prayer experience while waiting for a traffic light). Nurses can take advantage of passing moments to be still, be aware (Watson, 1999). Saidel (1996) offers several "tools for finding spirit and peace right where you are," including:

- Focusing on the present moment
- Forgiving and releasing yourself and others when grievances occur
- Being receptive to and trusting in the inner voice
- Treating others as we would like to be treated
- Letting go and moving on from things that you can no longer help
- Striving to be both nonoffensive and nondefensive
- Serving and encouraging others

Another way to cultivate spiritual self-awareness as a health care professional, according to Sulmasy (1999), is to deepen one's spiritual life within a religious tradition. Because religion is a bridge to spirituality and an expression of one's spirituality (see Chapter 1), it is logical that rooting oneself firmly within a religion can enhance personal spirituality. Cusveller (1995) argues that religious commitment provides religious nurses with a framework for determining the goals and purposes of their practice. Although religiousness can introduce bias and result in unethical spiritual care, as this chapter will later explore, it also can help nurses to become self-aware, spiritually aware.

Rew (2000) identifies several interventions for fostering self-awareness. Because these are also interventions a nurse can propose to a client, most are discussed in more detail elsewhere in this book. Rew recommends:

 - Keeping journals and diaries (see Chapter 11)
- Creating works of art—for example, knitting, sculpting, creating a flower garden (see Chapter 11)

- Writing letters to express feelings towards others. The letter can be edited and sent or shredded. Either way, the experience can be cathartic.
- Keeping an intuition log to record "ahas," hunches, and the "still small voice"
- Learning from dreams (see Chapter 11)
- Sharing stories, reminiscing, and conducting a life review (see Chapter 11)

Nagai-Jacobson and Burkhardt (1989) categorize activities that foster spirituality, referring to them as "Attending to That Which You Know," suggesting that these activities promote self-awareness. Grouped within the themes of connecting, disconnecting, journeying, transforming, skill acquisition, and washing away, these activities are presented in Box 3-3.

Box 3-3. Activities for Increasing Self-Awareness

Theme	Definition	Activities
Connecting	Seeking contact with self, others, universe, Ultimate Other; helps us settle in and touch the earth, heaven, past, present, future, loved ones near and far away	T'ai chi, talking on phone, writing letters, old photographs, and rituals
Disconnecting	Letting go; helps in connecting in different and creative ways	Free-form meditation, free dance, abandoned laughter, and guided meditation
Journeying	Taking a journey in time and space, moving through space; not "running away" but a skill to take care of yourself	Walking, reading epic novels, and journaling

(continues)

Box 3-3. Activities for Increasing Self-Awareness *(continued)*		
Theme	**Definition**	**Activities**
Transforming	Using raw materials to create something new and different or restoring order from chaos	Weaving, gardening, cleaning drawers, balancing a checkbook, and creative cooking
Skill acquisition	"Logical" problem solving or taking care of it by acquiring new skills	Taking a class and consulting a therapist
Washing away	Purifying, not necessarily with water	Showering or bathing, fasting, sitting before a fire, deep breathing, and gardening to "play in the dirt" rather than to transform the garden

Source: Adapted from Nagai-Jacobson, M. G., & Burkhardt, M. A. (1989). Spirituality: Cornerstone of holistic nursing practice. *Holistic Nursing Practice, 3*(3), 18–26. Reprinted by permission of Sage Publications, Inc.

Another method for building self-awareness is to take a self-assessment survey using a quantitative instrument (e.g., Dossey & Keegan [2000]). Other tools, such as the spiritual assessment form for clients found in Chapter 5 or research instruments that measure spiritual well-being, may be useful.

NURSING IMPLICATIONS

Sharing Spiritual Beliefs

The degree to which nurses are self-aware influences their nursing care, especially their spiritual caregiving. A nurse who has developed spiritual self-awareness will be better able to determine approaches that will serve to promote a client's spiritual well-being. Nurses who are aware of the influence of their religious or spiritual beliefs on their personal and professional lives will likely be more sensitive and careful when discussing spirituality or religion with clients. Conversely, a nurse with a poor understanding of how his or her beliefs may influence practice can potentially offend or distress clients. Understanding when it is or is not appropriate for the nurse to share personal religious and spiritual beliefs with clients is an important component of effective spiritual care.

Some clients will be comforted when a nurse shares spiritual beliefs; others may become annoyed and experience a loss of confidence in the nurse. It is also possible that a nurse can share spiritual beliefs in an inappropriate manner and thereby inflict spiritual distress (as defined in Chapter 1). It is this possibility that has led some to argue that health care professionals should never discuss spirituality with clients (Sloan et al., 2000). Because of the inevitability of clients' raising spiritual issues with nurses and the potential for healing that sharing spiritual beliefs can afford, the remainder of this chapter explores the issue of when and how it is appropriate to share personal beliefs with clients.

Consider the following scenarios recounted by oncology nurses:

> After a patient died, his daughter was having a difficult time. It had been a long illness, but she had been in denial until the end. In an appropriate moment, I said, "He went back to God who made him." After a minute, she asked, "What did you say?" I repeated my statement, and she seemed to get great comfort.

> The patient told me that the doctor said she didn't have much time and she should get her life in order. She was upset because she had been planning a trip in two years' time and now she wouldn't be able to go. She wasn't ready to die and was asking about what happened after life. I explained my belief that life on earth was just bearable and that life after death would be glorious and much better than life on earth. I suggested she remember that after death she'd be whole and pain free. I also suggested she ask God for guidance and grace.

In both of these scenarios, the nurse has made statements based on personal belief. Although the nurses imply that their spiritual care was effective, we can't confirm whether or not it was without knowing how their clients felt about hearing their words. If the clients in the above situations did not share beliefs similar to those of their nurses, it could be said that these nurses acted in such a way as to impose their beliefs on the clients. Although their intention to offer comfort was likely sincere, their methods may therefore have been inappropriate.

These scenarios raise many questions: How does a nurse discuss spiritual or religious beliefs while respecting the individuality and unique life perspective of the client? Although willfully imposing or forcing beliefs on a client clearly seems unethical, might purposeful withholding of helpful beliefs—or avoidance and disengagement about spiritual matters likewise be unethical? Certainly, there must be some middle ground from which a nurse can discuss spiritual beliefs in an ethical manner.

Applying recognized ethical principles provides a basis for establishing this middle ground. Ethics (see Chapter 1) studies human values and obligations. Several ethical principles to guide spiritual care include (Kozier, Erb, Berman, & Burke, 2000):

- Beneficence (doing good for clients)
- Nonmaleficence (doing no harm to clients)
- Autonomy (respecting and supporting others' rights to self-determination)
- Justice (or fairness)
- Fidelity (or faithfulness to previous agreements)
- Veracity (or truthtelling)

Thus, when considering whether to share spiritual beliefs with a client, the nurse should consider: Will revealing something about my own beliefs do good for or be harmful to my client? Will sharing my beliefs be respectful of my client's need to determine his or her own spiritual beliefs? Is sharing beliefs fair considering the possibly fragile spiritual state of the client? Would I be truthful if a client asked me about my beliefs and I choose not to respond?

Risk Factors

One factor that increases the risk of unethical spiritual care is the vulnerability of the client. Clients (as well as their families) are usually vulnerable by virtue of their illness or health challenge. Their vulnerability is physical, psychosocial, and spiritual. For example, a man recently diagnosed with multiple sclerosis faces physical limitations that will affect his ability to function socially. He may also be wondering "Why me?" and experiencing God as silent or absent. He may be starved for answers and meaning, leaving him spiritually vulnerable.

Another factor that increases risk for unethical spiritual caregiving exists when the nurse and client enter into an asymmetric relationship.

Nurses are socialized to behave from an interventionist framework. That is, they perceive themselves as more knowledgeable and thus more powerful than their clients. These perceptions may create an asymmetric relationship between clients and those professionals who care for them. This imbalance may allow the imposition of clinician beliefs on their clients (Mayer, 1992). An asymmetric relationship is manifested in statements nurses begin with phrases such as those presented in Box 3-4. A more symmetric relationship is indicated by the corresponding phrases.

In addition to client vulnerability and asymmetric relationships, other factors contribute to the potential for unethical spiritual caregiving. Nuances of these factors are revealed when exploring why clients ask nurses about their beliefs and why nurses sometimes share them.

"Nurse, What Do You Believe?"

Clients on occasion ask their nurses what they believe for a number of reasons. They may want information to aid their search for answers to spiritual questions. They may wish to gain a sense of whether the nurse is someone to whom it will be safe to disclose spiritual beliefs. Because clients often prefer to talk with someone with similar beliefs, they may check to see if the nurse shares similar views. Some clients may ask nurses about their beliefs in an attempt to establish or maintain a symmet-

Box 3-4. Phrases That Indicate Relationship Symmetry

Asymmetric (Inappropriate Phrase)	Symmetric (Appropriate phrase)
"Here, take this. . . ."	"Would you like to receive. . . ?"
"I need to teach you about. . . ."	"What would you like to learn about?"
"What I am doing for you will make you feel better."	"How can I help you to feel better?"
"You should do. . . ."	"May I make a suggestion?"

rical relationship. Others may question their nurse about spirituality to reciprocate the gift of listening that the nurse has given them—not to be a burden but to return the nurse's caring.

Although there is as of yet no research to document why nurses disclose personal spiritual beliefs with clients, it is possible to conjecture. Sensitive nurses characteristically are motivated to share personal spiritual beliefs with patients because of their sincere desire to provide spiritual comfort. It is hard to imagine that a caring nurse who is satisfied with his or her personal explanations for suffering would refuse to offer these explanations to a client coping with suffering and pleading for answers. Indeed, nurses often encounter clients at those times when they most crave spiritual comfort.

Another reason nurses disclose personal beliefs may arise from their recognition of the need to model the ability to express beliefs openly. Or the nurse may recognize, as Jourard (1964) reminds us, that self-disclosure begets self-disclosure and thus may choose self-disclosure as a method to encourage the client to disclose.

Proselytization, or the sharing of religious beliefs with others with the intent to convert them to a specific way of believing, can be viewed as existing along a continuum. At one end of this continuum is the ethical sharing of beliefs (i.e., in response to a specific client request), while the unethical imposition of beliefs on a vulnerable person reflects the other end (i.e., stating beliefs when a client asks that religion not be discussed). If a nurse unwittingly imposes beliefs without an express intent to proselytize, this act might fall in the middle of the continuum. Nurses, particularly those from evangelical and fundamental religious orientations, may feel a sense of obligation to inform clients about their perception of religious truth. This proselytization (or evangelism) reflects a compassionate desire on the part of the nurse to address the client's salvation. Especially when the client's death appears imminent, such evangelism may emerge.

When considering why clients may ask nurses about their spiritual beliefs and why nurses might disclose their spiritual beliefs, the potential for incongruency is evident. It is likely that a client who inquires about the nurse's beliefs in order to conduct a safety check and receives an evangelical response will not receive appropriate spiritual care. Or curious about the nurse's background, a client attempts to establish symmetry in the nurse–client relationship by striking up a conversation. This client's social needs may not be met, however, if the nurse chooses to share personal beliefs in an attempt to provide spiritual comfort.

Guidelines for Self-Disclosure

To what extent should a nurse express personal spiritual beliefs? What principles can guide nursing practice in this regard? Determining when and how much to disclose requires careful consideration. The following guidelines, drawn from several disciplines including nursing, ethics, and theology can help nurses to define the middle ground along the continuum that exists between ethical sharing of personal beliefs and unethical proselytization. (Principles of empathic listening, presented in Chapter 4, can also help the nurse to determine appropriate levels of disclosure.)

Establish Nurse–Client Boundaries

Knowledge about the appropriate use of self-disclosure helps to establish a therapeutic relationship with a client. Wilson and Kneisl (1996) define self-disclosure as "being open to personal feelings and experiences, being 'real' as opposed to hiding behind a professional facade" (p. 680). They present this concept as a continuum from underdisclosure to overdisclosure suggesting that nurses can disclose too much or too little about their personal beliefs. To help a nurse determine whether a given level of self-disclosure is appropriate, prior to self-disclosure, the nurse can ask:

- What is the purpose of my self-revelation? For whom is this disclosure?
- Will my disclosure enhance a therapeutic relationship?

The nurse will benefit by evaluating the effectiveness of the disclosure. Was the self-revelation facilitative? If unsure, he or she may ask the patient, "How did you feel when I told you about my personal beliefs?" The nurse may also consider prefacing any self-disclosure of spiritual beliefs with a caveat such as "I know you asked me about my beliefs, but I don't want to impose them on you in any way that might not be helpful to you."

If the nurse senses that self-disclosure would not be therapeutic, the client's request for self-disclosure can be deflected with one of the techniques presented in Box 3-5. It is important to note, however, that ethical spiritual caregiving does not always require deflecting requests for self-disclosure. Indeed, more often than not, it may call for careful and appropriate sharing of personal beliefs.

Box 3-5. Techniques for Deflecting Requests for Self-Disclosure

Use honesty (e.g., "I am sensing that it would be best to not share my personal beliefs with you at this time.")

Use benign curiosity (e.g., "I wonder why you're asking me this?")

Use refocusing (e.g., "You were telling me about how you wondered 'Why me, God?' I wonder why you turned your question around to me. Can you take some time now and think about your answer?")

Seek clarification (e.g., "You keep asking me about my own beliefs about what happens after death. I wonder what concerns you might be having about me?")

Respond with feedback and limit-setting (e.g., "I think it is possibly inappropriate for me to share my personal beliefs with you. Talking about my religion isn't appropriate for our relationship.")

Practice Existential Advocacy

Nurses ought to try to balance respect for client autonomy with recognition of the professional expertise they have to offer. Paternalistic attempts to influence client spiritual beliefs may be just as inappropriate as remaining completely uninvolved. A caring and aware involvement that reflects respect for the individual is appropriate. Gadow (1990) called this middle ground "existential advocacy."

Examine Your Motivation

As Wilson and Kneisl (1996) suggested, nurses should ask themselves what prompts them to reveal personal spiritual beliefs. If disclosure serves to meet the needs of the nurse rather than those of the client, then it is likely to be inappropriate.

Strive for Symmetry in Client Relationships

Efforts to achieve symmetry in a relationship with a vulnerable client are enhanced when nurses are aware of their own vulnerabilities. When nurses acknowledge their own spiritual struggles, doubts, questions, and insecurities, they will encounter clients from a place of shared woundedness. As discussed earlier in this chapter, those who see themselves as "wounded healers" are often the most effective healers.

Respond in Ways That Strengthen Nurse–Client Relationships

Nurses who listen with empathy and have determined what motivates a client to ask about their spiritual beliefs will be able to respond in a manner that enhances the nurse–client relationship. For example, a nurse may preface a response with, "I am happy to answer your question about what I believe, but I don't want to do it in a way that is imposing. Please tell me if I talk too much!" The nurse can also be careful to respond with brief statements, allowing clients to probe further if they desire. Commenting about one's spiritual beliefs without disparaging other ways of believing is also appropriate. If the nurse has any doubt about the appropriateness of his or her self-disclosure, a follow-up question may prove helpful.

Observe the Golden Rule

"Do unto others as you would have them do unto you." This and similar proverbs, which are common to various cultural groups and belief systems, can help the nurse to gauge the appropriateness of disclosing personal beliefs. Nurses can ask themselves, "If I were in this client's situation, would I want to hear my nurse say what I want to say now?"

Offer Responses That Reflect a Common Ground

When client beliefs differ from those of the nurse, and the client has not expressed a desire for information about other beliefs, the nurse can share spiritual beliefs that are sufficiently universal to be comforting. The nurse who is able to reflect shared foundational beliefs creates a broader framework in which nurse and client will find unity. A Christian nurse and a Muslim patient, for example, can agree that they seek comfort from a Divine Being though they may choose to label this Being differently. An agnostic nurse and a Jewish client may agree that seeking love and peace for all people is a primary goal and motivator. Other nurse–client dyads that encompass different worldviews may share the idea that finding meaning in suffering is desirable but difficult, that there is an afterlife of some sort, or that there is an Inner Light that guides them.

Understanding whether, when, and how to share personal beliefs requires self-awareness and spiritual assessment skills (see Chapter 5). A nurse must be honest and sensitive about what motivates him or her to share spiritual beliefs with clients. Even nurses who have developed a high degree of self-awareness must assess the appropriateness of sharing beliefs before doing so. Box 3-6 presents one nurse's approach to finding appropriate ways to offer spiritual support.

Box 3-6. One Nurse's Story

Patricia Marsella, RN, MSN, an oncology nurse on Long Island, New York, shares how self-awareness influences her nursing care:

To enter into a therapeutic relationship which encourages a dialogue about the spiritual dimension for the benefit of patient wellness, a number of assumptions, techniques, and guidelines are required. Foremost, this is not an avenue for me to convince anyone that the God of my understanding needs to be the God of their experience. An underlying assumption here might be that to provide spiritual care for another, the nurse must have a clearly defined sense and experience of God—God being a deity, force, supreme being, or simply "Good Orderly Direction" that enlivens and gives one's life meaning and purpose. This assumption is not necessarily true.

A nurse who lacks faith or belief can foster a dialogue with a patient about spiritual concerns just as easily as one who has great faith and con-viction. The point is that the nurse's level of spiritual pursuit or develop-ment does not determine the help a patient may receive in her or his per-sonal journey. What is needed is an awareness of and an ability to dialogue about that which is spiritual.

Mr. K and I shared a wonderful therapeutic relationship that spanned years. Mr. K claimed to be Roman Catholic. I was interested in what that meant to him as he seemed to be struggling to understand the "why's" of his illness. He also expressed concern as to how he could help his family cope with his terminal condition. He admitted after some dialogue that he had one little problem with Catholicism. He wasn't quite sure if Jesus was God!

I smiled and said, "Hey, Mr. K, I'd say you have more than a little problem if you don't believe Jesus is God. My understanding of Catholicism is that that is the whole ball of wax." He laughed and remarked that he was amazed to be talking about these matters with me. Even his wife did not know the dilemma in his mind.

My demeanor was professional, yet because of our nurse–client relationship I knew I could joke in this manner with Mr. K. I attempted to highlight his concern, to respect his view, and not try to convince him of anything. I asked if he wanted to see a clergyperson to talk about this matter, but he declined.

Mr. K asked me what I believed. In a therapeutic relationship, self-disclo-sure can be a powerful tool that shows the nurse to be human, caring, and nonjudgmental. The judicious, deliberate use of self-disclosure can help a patient feel accepted and understood and can normalize an experience or emotion that is painful, shame producing, or overwhelming. Disclosure may

Box 3-6. One Nurse's Story *(continued)*

also help a patient clarify beliefs or decisions. I am not interested in "enlightening" a person, but respect that each person is on a personal spiritual path directed by God. Each person responds to God individually based on background, tradition, circumstances, and beliefs. One of my roles is to enhance or contribute to patients' spiritual wellness as they follow their spiritual path.

KEY POINTS

- Self-awareness is essential for nurses if they are to be healers or effective spiritual care providers.
- Being, as well as doing, is an important component of spiritual care.
- Nursing research demonstrates that the degree to which nurses consider themselves spiritual influences their attitude toward spiritual care and their comfort with providing such care.
- Practical suggestions for developing self-awareness include finding safe individuals and situations for sharing feelings, keeping journals and logs, creating art, and making sense of dreams, and attending more seriously to one's religion.
- Nurses, often unwittingly, can impose their spiritual or religious beliefs on clients.
- Client vulnerability and characteristic asymmetrical nurse–client relationships contribute to the risk for inappropriate self-disclosure of spiritual beliefs.
- Responses to client questions about the nurse's personal beliefs are most effective when congruent with the client's reasons for asking.
- Guidelines for nurses to determine whether and how to disclose personal spiritual beliefs include: considering one's motivation to disclose, observing the "golden rule," and seeking common ground.

LOOK WITHIN TO LEARN

1. Complete the self-assessment presented in Box 3-1. What might you do to increase your effectiveness as a healer (considering the suggestions in Box 3-3)?

2. How would you characterize your spiritual health? To what degree are you spiritually aware? How will this influence the nursing care you provide?

3. What are the reasons that you share your beliefs (in general or about spirituality) with others? Is it because you are excited by your beliefs? Is it because you want others to think the way you do? Would you be uncomfortable being around someone who believes in a way different from you? Why or why not?

4. Consider this observation made by a nursing student:

   One day in the hospital, I saw an RN slip a prayer card in between the fingers of a patient as he was preparing to go down for surgery. To the best of my knowledge, the patient had not indicated a belief in God. The patient and his family seemed uncomfortable when this happened. Later, I asked the RN why she did this, and she told me that this is what she did for all of her patients.

   Was this nurse providing sensitive, effective spiritual care? Why or why not? What techniques might you use to determine whether or not this care was appropriate? If you were a colleague, what would you say or do if you felt that the nurse had acted inappropriately?

REFERENCES

(**Bold** print indicates those that are most recommended.

Boutell, K. A., & Bozett, F. W. (1987). Nurses' assessment of patients' spirituality: Continuing education implications. *Journal of Continuing Education in Nursing, 21,* 172–176.

Brittain, J. N. (1986). Theological foundations for spiritual care. *Journal of Religion and Health, 25,* 107–121.

Cusveller, B. S. (1995). A view from somewhere: The presence and function of religious commitment in nursing practice. *Journal of Advanced Nursing, 22,* 973–978.

Danvers, M. A. (1998). Keeping in good spirits. *Nursing Management, 5*(5), 35–37.

Dominic, A. P. (1988, September). A natural principle of spirituality. *Review for Religious,* 748–754.

Dossey, B. M., & Keegan, L. (2000). Self-assessments: Facilitating healing in self and others. In B. M. Dossey, L. Keegan, & C. E. Guzzetta (Eds.), *Holistic nursing: A handbook for practice* (3rd ed., Chapter 15, pp. 361–374). Rockville, MD: Aspen.

Dossey, B. M., Keegan, L., & Guzzetta, C. E. (Eds.). (2000). *Holistic nursing: A handbook for practice* (3rd ed). Rockville, MD: Aspen.

Gadow, S. (1990). Existential advocacy: Philosophical foundations of nursing. In T. Pence et al. (Eds.), *Ethics in nursing: An anthology* (pp. 41–51). National League for Nursing Publication 20-2294.

Highfield, M. E. F., Taylor, E. J., & Amenta, M. O. (2000). "Preparation to care: The spiritual care education of oncology and hospice nurses. *Journal of Hospice & Palliative Nursing, 2*(2), 53–63.

Jourard, S. (1964). *The transparent self: Self disclosure and well being.* New York: Van Nostrand, Reinhold.

Kozier, B., Erb, G., Berman, A. J., & Burke, K. (2000). *Fundamentals of nursing: Concepts, process, and practice (6th ed.).* Upper Saddle River, NJ: Prentice Hall Health.

Mayer, J. (1992). Wholly responsible for a part, or partly responsible for a whole? The concept of spiritual care in nursing. *Second Opinion, 17*(3), 26–55.

McKivergin, M. (2000). The nurse as an instrument of healing. In B. M. Dossey, L. Keegan, & C. E. Guzzetta (Eds.), *Holistic nursing: A handbook for practice* (3rd ed., Chapter 10, pp. 207–228). Rockville, MD: Aspen.

Millison, M. B., & Dudley, J. R. (1992). Providing spiritual support: A job for all hospice professionals. *Hospice Journal, 8*(4), 49–66.

Nagai-Jacobson, M. G., & Burkhardt, M. A. (1989). Spirituality: Cornerstone of holistic nursing practice. *Holistic Nursing Practice, 3*(3), 18–26.

Nouwen, H. J. M. (1979). *The wounded healer.* Garden City, NJ: Image Books.

Piles, C. (1990). Providing spiritual care. *Nurse Educator, 15*(1), 36–41.

Quinn, J. (2000). Transpersonal human caring and healing. In B. M. Dossey, L. Keegan, & C. E. Guzzetta (Eds.), *Holistic nursing: A handbook for practice* (3rd ed., Chapter 2, pp. 37–48). Rockville, MD: Aspen.

Rew, L. (2000). Self-reflection: Consulting the truth within. In B. M. Dossey, L. Keegan, & C. E. Guzzetta (Eds.), *Holistic nursing: A handbook for practice* (3rd ed., Chapter 17, pp. 407–424). Rockville, MD: Aspen.

Ross, L. A. (1994). Spiritual aspects of nursing. *Journal of Advanced Nursing, 19,* 439–447.

Saidel, I. G. (1996). Finding spirituality at work: A strategy for challenging times. *Aspen's Advisor for Nurses Executives, 11*(4), 7–8.

Sloan, R. P., Bagiella, E., VandeCreek, L., Hover, M., Casalone, C., Hirsch, T. J., Hasan, Y., Kreger, R., & Poulos, P. (2000). Should physicians prescribe religious activities? *New England Journal of Medicine, 342,* 1913–1916.

Soeken, K., & Carson, V. B. (1986, April). Study measures nurses' attitudes about providing spiritual care. *Health Progress,* 52–55.

Sulmasy, D. P. (1999). Is medicine a spiritual practice? *Academic Medicine, 74,* 1002–1004.

Taylor, E. J., Highfield, M., & Amenta, M. (1994). Attitudes and beliefs regarding spiritual care: A survey of cancer nurses. *Cancer Nursing, 17*(6), 479–487.

Taylor, E. J., Highfield, M. F., & Amenta, M. O. (1999). Predictors of oncology and hospice nurses' spiritual care perspectives and practices. *Applied Nursing Research, 12*(1), 30—37.

Watson, J. (1999). Becoming aware: Knowing yourself to care for others. *Home health care Nurse, 17,* 317–322.

Wilson, H. S., & Kneisl, C. R. (1996). *Psychiatric nursing* (5th ed.). Menlo Park, CA: Addison-Wesley.

Part II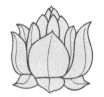

Nursing the Spirit:
Application to Practice

4

Communicating Support for Spiritual Health

Imagine yourself as a client with a challenging health problem who feels afraid and alone. Perhaps you are about to undergo surgery or are enduring uncontrolled pain. Would you wish for someone to be there for you? Someone trustworthy who seemed to understand what you were experiencing? Someone who could help you make sense of your thoughts and feelings? For most, the answer is "yes!"

The ability to communicate compassionate support is a fundamental nursing skill essential to the process of promoting spiritual health. This chapter explores aspects of communication, including verbal, nonverbal, and presencing that are considered most useful by spiritual care providers. Effective use of these approaches enables nurses to establish trust, exude calmness, and convey joy, as well as to provide companionship and other elemental gifts that serve to inspirit clients.

FORMS OF COMMUNICATION

Verbal Communication: Listening and Speaking

Active, empathic listening, key to spiritual caregiving, nurtures spiritual health. Listening is an essential element of nursing activities that promote spiritual health, including conducting a spiritual assessment, helping clients to make meaning of their suffering, and planning spiritual rituals.

After synthesizing the nursing literature about listening, Fredriksson (1999) concluded that active, empathic, or therapeutic listening is characterized by the following attributes: intentional inner silencing, focusing, and concentration by the listener; attentiveness to nonverbal and verbal messages from the sender, including vocal tone, pitch, and speed; allowance of time for the communicators to express their story; and listener reflection and interpretation, which is offered as feedback to promote the speaker's understanding. Listening at this level requires energy and skill and contributes to a caring relationship in which clients feel "heard."

Levels of Empathic Listening

Multiple levels of empathic listening exist. Rowan (1986) proposed that individuals listen at four levels:

- **Basic Accurate Empathy.** At the most basic level, listener and speaker interact intellect to intellect. The listener is able to play back what the speaker has said in such a way that the speaker recognizes it.
- **Advanced Accurate Empathy.** At this level, feelings as well as intellect are aligned. The listener incorporates emotional aspects of what was heard in the response constructed for the client; this feedback helps the client feel understood and accepted.
- **Awareness.** The third level of listening finds the listener aware of the client's physical as well as emotional and intellectual messages. The nurse notes the client's posture, gestures, movements, breathing, and voice quality. Even the way in which clients position themselves (e.g., sitting behind a desk, placing a pillow in front of them) may be important. Nurse responses to client messages incorporate this awareness (e.g., "Mrs. Lee, as I heard you talk about the embarrassment of living with your disability, I noticed your jaws tighten. Can you tell me what that might mean?"). Listeners at this level also tune into *their* inner physical feelings generated in response to the client.

- **Advanced Awareness.** At this level, the listener is aware of the speaker's thoughts, feelings, bodily expressions, and spirituality. Rowan referred to this level as holistic listening and as being "aware of our experience in the ever-flowing present" (p. 90). A holistic listener uses intuition and maintains an awareness of the transpersonal or something greater than the self to make insightful responses. A holistic listener is aware of the "holy" in the encounter.

Guidelines for Empathic Listening

There is a misconception that empathic listening is natural and easy. On the contrary, it is a skill that requires sensitivity and practice and extends beyond fundamental listening techniques (e.g., asking open-ended questions and using summarization, clarification, paraphrasing, etc.). Key aspects of listening empathically to promote spiritual health are:

- Striving to hear all aspects of the client's message
- Recognizing your inner response
- Helping clients to listen to themselves and make sense from what they have heard

Hearing the Client

The goal of empathic listening is a therapeutic one. The nurse distinguishes between therapeutic and social interactions (Fortinash & Holoday-Worret, 2000), focusing on the client's needs and refraining from using conversation to meet personal needs. An indication that empathic listening is occurring is revealed by who does most of the talking. An empathic listener with a therapeutic goal may talk less than 5 to 10 percent of the time; thus, it is the client who speaks most.

Myers's (2000) in-depth interviews with recipients of psychotherapy revealed several factors that make a client feel truly heard. Empathic therapists:
- Allowed clients to hear themselves
- Did not "flinch" when clients expressed various pains
- Made clients feel accepted, even while aware of their undesirable characteristics
- Helped clients to make sense of their own confusion
- Made clients feel that their stories were valuable
- Provided feedback to clients (e.g., by asking questions and paraphrasing or summarizing their comments)

Myers concluded that what makes a therapist ultimately effective is the quality of the connection built between the client and therapist.

Balzer-Riley (1996) identified additional points for nurses to consider when listening empathically. In addition to clearing distracting agendas from one's mind and focusing on the speaker, Balzer-Riley advised that nurses reflect on what the client wants them to hear. For example, clients who describe themselves as very religious and take great effort to list all the religious activities in which they have been involved may want the nurse to perceive them as pious. Such behavior may indicate the need for respect and could also suggest the need to disguise reality.

Recognizing the Inner Response

The way a nurse responds to a client is drawn not only from a client's messages but also intuitive or "gut" feelings. Rowan (1986) suggested that feelings that emerge in the listener may mirror the true feelings of the client. An angry client, for instance, who may even deny feeling angry, may make a nurse inwardly feel tense or angry. Often, individuals somatize the feelings they witness with tension in the neck and shoulders, "goose bumps," a tightness in the chest, or a sense that the "stomach is in knots." Being attentive to these inner feelings can alert a nurse to a client's true emotions, sometimes before they arise in the verbal conversation.

Helping the Client to be Heard

"Naming the silences" is an approach to responding to spiritual pain that helps clients to hear and make sense of their suffering (Hauerwas, 1990). Acknowledging spiritual pain requires strength, and repressing it may exacerbate suffering. Thus, by assisting clients to acknowledge spiritual distress, the nurse helps to free them from its crippling effects. Therapeutic phrases like "We feel purposeless when we feel we are a burden to others," or "It is not unusual to feel betrayed when someone seems to have broken unspoken rules" (i.e., "We feel _____ when _____") are examples of how a nurse can assist the client to name a silent spiritual pain.

Silence, an inevitable part of conversational flow, allows clients to hear themselves. Rybarczyk and Bellg (1997) emphasized the importance of permitting moments of silence to occur during client interactions. Silence has several functions. It allows clients to gather their thoughts without being interrupted. Meaningful thoughts do take time to be formulated; they also take time to be recollected from old memories. A nurse who respects silences communicates to clients that they are "center stage," they may proceed with their story at their own pace, and they don't have to continue talking just to keep the nurse present. Rybarczyk and Bellg observed that the most significant statements of a conversation will often occur right after a period of silence.

Clients who have truly been heard both by the nurse and themselves exhibit a somatic expression of release. This may be an "aha!", a heavy sigh, or shedding tears. The empathic nurse does not flinch or indicate discomfort with tears or any other manifestation of client emotion. Tears have been considered by spiritual mystics as kisses of God, or a special gift that cleanses. Nurses can assist clients to appreciate the healing value of tears by responding respectfully when they happen. In some circumstances, the nurse may find crying with a client to be mutually therapeutic.

Nonverbal Communication

Communication that effectively promotes spiritual health requires the nurse to recognize and respond to client nonverbal as well as verbal messages. Nonverbal communication, in continual use by conscious persons, generally provides more accurate information about emotions than does verbal communication. Nonverbal communication includes touch, body movements, facial expressions, gestures, posture and gait, and even the way people dress or otherwise decorate themselves. Because touch has historically often been associated with spiritual healing, it will be discussed here along with a brief summary of messages communicated by other forms of body language.

Touch

Touch can be a powerful method for communicating support and nurturing spiritual health. Touch is often categorized in nursing literature (Estabrooks & Morse, 1992; Fredriksson, 1999) as:

- Procedural touch (touch necessary to perform tasks such as measuring vital signs)
- Nonprocedural touch (or comforting, nonnecessary, positive affective touch)
- Protective touch (a means for the nurse, via a cold or harsh touch, to find emotional protection by distancing from a client or releasing tension)

Although the effect of touch on the spiritual health of clients has not been directly studied, empirical evidence indicates that comforting touch can contribute to positive client outcomes that may be related to improved spiritual health. That is, caring touch has been observed to decrease patient anxiety and psychological distress, to enhance self-esteem, and to increase a sense of security, feelings of connectedness and acceptance, and the degree of self-disclosure to nurses (Fredriksson, 1999; Weiss, 1986).

Factors Determining Client Responses

Weiss (1986) observed many factors that determine client response to a nurse's caring touch. These include the client's previous experiences of touch, culture, personal views about what is appropriate touch, gender (and gender of the nurse touching), age, and physical health status. Although research suggests these factors influence response to touch, there is not enough evidence to state specific predictive relationships that could guide nursing practice. This evidence does, however, inform nurses to be sensitive to possible factors that influence client responses to touch.

After reviewing touch research, Weiss (1986) also observed that client perceptions of the intent of a nurse's touch may be a major factor that determines the therapeutic value of the outcome. If the nurse provides procedural or nonprocedural touch with the intent to comfort, then the client will likely have a positive response. In contrast, if the nurse provides touch, even a simple pat on the hand, without a genuine intent to comfort, the client may perceive this incongruent message and not respond positively.

Guidelines for Touching

How a nurse touches a client greatly determines the outcome of touch. Nurses must be vigilant about their attitudes toward their clients and their work. An attitude of caring promotes effective touching whether the situation is nonprocedural or procedural. Imagine the client response to the nurse who provides a bedbath with resentment or irritation as compared to the nurse who views this task as an opportunity for loving service.

In addition to qualitative features of touch (e.g., lightness, length, and manner), it is important to consider where to touch clients. The limbs of the body are generally considered more appropriate places to offer caring touch. Because the torso represents the core of the body, clients may perceive this area as too intimate for touch other than procedural. The wrist and forearm are usually excellent areas to touch to communicate comfort. If the client offers a hand, handholding can also be comforting.

Conveying superiority or power while touching does not express caring and can be avoided by refraining from:

- Giving pats on the back, which may be perceived as belittling
- Touching the shoulders while standing over the client in a way that implies "I'm more powerful than you"
- Gripping the upper arm while holding hands in a way that implies, "I'm keeping you in your place" (When holding hands or touching the forearm, it may be best to place the client's arm or hand on top; in effect, the nurse's hands can cradle and support the client.)

Nurses sometimes fear that clients may misinterpret their touch as a sexual overture and thus may withhold touch when it might be therapeutic. It is less likely that a client will misinterpret if the nurse touches at an appropriate time and place and with a nonsexual intent. Asking for permission may clarify intent (e.g., "I can see that this is a rough time for you. Would having me hold your hand be comforting?").

Box 4-1 illustrates the power of caring touch, even when it begins as procedural touch.

Body Language

Effective communication requires that nurses be cognizant not only of client body language, but also their own body language. Body language reveals much about a client's emotional state. Conversely, body language informs clients about how sincere, interested, and receptive a nurse is toward them.

Considerations that can guide the nurse to interpret body language include:

- What are the client's eyes communicating? Do they shift nervously? Do they avoid connecting?
- What do other facial messages suggest? Does the face "light up" or look tired?
- How does the client position his or her body? Tilted away to create distance? Arms crossed to create a barrier?
- How does the client use furniture, clothing, or other objects to communicate? Does the client, for example, hold an object closely like a shield?
- What might the quality of the voice indicate? Is it high and tight with fright, or fast with worry?
- What do the client's gestures indicate? Is there a nervous fidgeting?

When considering such elements of communication, it is essential that the nurse be sensitive to the presence of gender, age, social, and cultural variations. An Asian client, for example, may avoid eye contact but focus instead on the nurse's chin to show respect.

Nurses should also consider what their body language communicates during interactions with clients. When discussing a spiritual topic

---

Box 4-1. One Nurse's Story: The Power of Touch

Martel Costa, RN, BSN, worked as an aide in a urban community hospital at the time she had this experience:

The surgical step-down unit was very busy the day I had an unforgettable experience with a client. Mrs. P, an Armenian woman in her late 50s, spoke no English. During my shift, she had no visitors and seemed sad and withdrawn. In the afternoon, I went to her room and, using hand motions, asked her if she was ready to be bathed. She nodded yes.

I began by carefully wiping her face. To me, touching the face is one of the most effective ways to provide nurturing. I gently wiped around her eyes and forehead. She began to relax and closed her eyes. I interpreted her behavior as an indication that she was enjoying the physical contact. So I continued to bathe her, moving from her face to her neck, and then to her back.

As I washed her back, Mrs. P began to cry softly. I became alarmed. Was I hurting her? She didn't appear to be in pain. She began to pray aloud, repeatedly thanking God. She seemed to need someone to reach out to her and care for her with compassion. I stopped the bath, and kneeling beside her, I held her hand.

She continued to cry. We looked at each other. I thought, "There is nothing I can say that she will understand." I sensed that my look conveyed much more than words could anyway. After a few minutes, I resumed bathing her. Because she had enjoyed the physical contact, I applied lotion to her back. The woman closed her eyes again, praying periodically as I rubbed her back.

Before I left that day, I went to Mrs. P's room to say good-bye. She took my hands and kissed them and repeatedly thanked me. I was touched that a small act like bathing could make such a difference. Despite a language barrier, I felt that we established a profound bond.

that the nurse may experience as embarrassing or painful, do fidgeting, nervous facial expressions, or inappropriate giggling occur? When inviting a client to talk about spiritual concerns, does the nurse pull up a chair and sit down, maintain eye contact, lean forward, and in other ways convey receptivity? Or does the nurse's body language communicate defensiveness, disinterest, or emotional distance?

Empathic responses incorporate reflection on and often mention of client nonverbal messages. To illustrate, a nurse might say: "While you were telling me about your family, I heard your voice sort of crack as though it was hurt" or "It looks to me like your eyes are looking off to a faraway place." Allow clients to validate such observations. Sometimes, it is best to ask clients to interpret their nonverbal messages (e.g., "I noticed _____. Can you tell me if that meant anything?").

Responding to Client Messages

A client's suffering and spiritual distress sometimes create discomfort for nurses regarding how to formulate a suitable response. Often, the most appropriate response is silence but sometimes a verbal response is also helpful. Pastoral counselor William Oglesby (1980), proposed a formula for creating helpful responses, "There you are; here I am; I love you." Nurses can apply this formula by responding in ways that convey recognition of the client's experience and the nurse's presence for the client and by closing with an indication that the nurse cares for the client. A nurse, for example, might adapt Oglesby's formula this way: "As I listen to you, I'm sensing your fear; I just want you to know that I care about what happens to you."

Rybarczyk and Bellg (1997) also advocate that the listener identify themes in the client's story (e.g., "It seems to me as I hear you speak that you see yourself as someone who has survived against great odds") or elements of the client's manner of speaking (e.g., "I am noticing that you are really animated when you talk about your religion"). Rybarczyk and Bellg suggest that the listener may want to mirror the speaker's gestures, if appropriate. By reflecting the client's thinking and feeling through gestures, the listener demonstrates awareness of the speaker's multimodal message.

Clients present a myriad of thoughts and feelings within a conversation. It can sometimes be difficult to discern what theme or content should be the focus of a response. Clues may be provided when the following are taken into consideration:

- Are there incongruencies between verbal and nonverbal messages?
- Where does the client place verbal or physical energy when talking? (e.g., What topic makes the client's eyes "brighten?" What is he or she talking about when speech increases in volume and speed?)
- What emotional undercurrents are present?
- What loaded words does the clients use?
- Are figures of speech used that indicate a topic is emphasized?

A summary of techniques to guide nurse responses to client messages is provided in Box 4-2.

PRESENCING

Being fully present for clients is an essential component of caring. It is especially important when caring for clients with spiritual needs. When nurses are queried about interventions they use to provide spiritual care, they typically include communication strategies that convey presence, like "active listening" and "just being there" (Emblen & Halstead, 1993; Sellers & Haag, 1998; Taylor, Amenta, & Highfield, 1995). Effective presencing requires authentic and expert use of verbal and nonverbal communication strategies.

Presencing, the translation of the noun "presence" into a verb denoting action, is a practice that nurses are beginning to appreciate as a clinical "intervention." Presencing—being present, being there, being with—is a term coined by Benner in the 1984 seminal book, *From Novice to Expert,* to identify one of the competencies incorporated by expert nurses in the helping role (Zerwekh, 1997). Several philosophers and nurse theorists identify and explain the need for presencing (Zerwekh). Although research exists that documents client and nurse appreciation for presencing, there is little empirical research that specifically describes it or its outcomes (Gardner, 1992; Minicucci, 1998).

Pettigrew (1990) identified distinguishing features of presencing. Elements that are unique to presencing include the following aspects of relating to another person:

- Giving of self in the present moment
- Being available with all of the self
- Listening, with full awareness of the privilege of doing so
- Being there in a way that is meaningful to another person

Box 4-2. Techniques for Empathic Listening

Do:
- Maintain an attitude of caring.
- Place full attention in the present moment and on the client to be present to clients in their deepest moments.
- Refrain from personal issues and stories.
- Attend to client feelings as well as thoughts.
- Attend to nonverbal messages as well as verbal messages.
- Be aware of inner responses to a client.
- Look for client indications of feeling heard (e.g., "Yeah, that's what I mean.")
- Use the client's terminology for concepts when formulating responses.
- Allow silence.
- Accept tears.
- Note the client's use of figures of speech and energy placement.
- Respect the client's desire for closeness *or distance* and use it for healing purposes.
- Integrate verbal and nonverbal client messages when forming responses
- Add up, reflect, and respond to what clients say in a way that allows clients to gain further understanding.

Don't:
- Tell your "counter story" unless you determine it to be therapeutic for the client.
- Change the topic of conversation to avoid emotional discomfort.
- "Sweep feelings under the carpet" or in any way minimize emotional discomforts.
- Impose positivity.
- Focus on tangential details or facts when it is the emotional response to a circumstance that the client needs to discuss.
- Assume an attitude of superiority or savior, e.g.: *"I know that everything will be alright."*
- Offer responses that preach or attempt to fix client emotional pain.

Presencing overlaps or is closely related to other concepts such as empathy, support, caring, listening, attending, communicating, and therapeutic use of self (Gardner, 1992). In an analysis of the concept of presence, Fredriksson (1999) noted that presencing is a "gift of self" given by the nurse who maintains an attitude of attentiveness for the client. Thus, nurses who listen attentively to clients yet fail to give of self (i.e., do not inwardly "make room") diminish their effectiveness (Minicucci, 1998; Pettigrew).

Some nurse authors have described presencing as having multiple levels (Fredriksson, 1999; Snyder, Brandt, & Tseng, 2000). Osterman and Schwartz-Barcott (1996) proposed four ways of being present for clients:

- *Presence*, as these authors define it, is exhibited when a nurse is physically present but not focused on the client. A nurse who watches television in a client's room with no interaction is an example.
- *Partial presence* is characterized by the nurse's being physically present and attending to some task on the client's behalf but without relating to the client on any but the most superficial level. Silently changing an intravenous catheter while thinking about a dinner party is an example.
- *Full presence* refers to mental, emotional, and physical presence. The nurse intentionally focuses on the client. A nurse who observes and listens fully to assist the client to problem solve is being fully present.
- *Transcendent presence* occurs when a nurse is physically, mentally, emotionally, and spiritually present for a client. This type of presence involves a transpersonal and transforming experience. A nurse practicing therapeutic touch, co-meditation, or prayer with a client would likely be providing a transcendent presence. So also would a nurse who silently and purposefully, intentionally, and wholeheartedly stays with a client in severe pain.

Dimensions of Presencing

How does one provide presence? Several scholars have sought to characterize the nature of presencing (Fredriksson, 1998; Gardner, 1992; Zerwekh, 1997), and Pettigrew (1990) identified four essential components of presencing: client vulnerability, silence, invitation, and privilege.

Client Vulnerability

Presencing is often the best and sometimes the only intervention to support a client who suffers under circumstances that medical interventions cannot address. When a client is helpless, powerless, and vulnerable, a nurse's presencing can be most beneficial. Observing another person who is suffering and helpless is incredibly challenging. It is a difficult realization for a health care professional to conclude that one's professional expertise can no longer cure or comfort a client. When confronted with such vulnerability, it is common to avoid it, or to protect oneself from it by using professional tactics (e.g., keeping busy with technical tasks or offering counsel). Pettigrew (1990) contends, however, that "vulnerability demands vulnerability in order to come alongside one who is suffering" (p. 505). Presencing requires that the nurse recognize the helplessness of the situation and yet remain amidst it. Rather than worrying about saying or doing "the right thing," the nurse focuses on being fully present.

Silence

Pettigrew (1990) refers to silence as the "language of suffering." Often, words are inadequate to express vulnerability and suffering. Words may even trivialize a painful experience. Presencing, therefore, often involves being with a client in silence. The nurse's silence is essential when a client pleads, "Will you please just listen?"

Invitation

Presencing requires an invitation from the client. Because many clients regard suffering as a private matter, it is imperative that the nurse obtain permission to witness and accompany clients in their vulnerable state. "The invitation is to come alongside and be allowed to see, to share, to touch, and to hear the brokenness, vulnerability, and suffering of another" (Pettigrew, 1990, p. 505).

Privilege

"Presence is always a privilege for a nurse, never a right" (Pettigrew, 1990, p. 505). It requires a great deal of courage for a client to reveal vulnerabilities, losses, and suffering because these could be met with a response that recoils from, minimizes, or denies those painful realities. Thus, when a client allows a nurse to be present to his or her suffering, the nurse should recognize this as a gift—a privilege—from the client.

Zerwekh (1997) recognized that presencing is not only a privilege for nurses, but that it can be an activity that brings comfort to the nurse. That is, by comforting others, the nurse gains a deeper sense of inner comfort.

Outcomes of Presencing

Positive outcomes of presencing identified by nurses (Fredriksson, 1999; Gardner, 1992; Osterman & Schwartz-Barcott, 1996; Snyder, Brandt, & Tseng, 2000) include:

- Diminished suffering
- Decreased anxiety
- Psychospiritual growth through challenging life experiences
- Decreased sense of isolation
- Increased sense of connectedness
- Increased sense of having been heard and cared for, comforted, and encouraged
- Opportunity to put thoughts and feelings into words
- Decreased sense of vulnerability
- Increased self-understanding and motivation

Osterman and Schwartz-Barcott (1996) identify negative outcomes that can occur when nurses offer presencing. For their presence and partial presence categories, missed opportunities for building relationship may contribute to client anxiety. The potential negative outcomes of full presencing, however, affect the nurse as well as the client. Osterman and Scharwarz-Barcott suggest that if nurses place too much energy into being present, a client may feel uncomfortable. With transcendent presencing, the nurse's objectivity may be compromised by fusing too closely with the client's experience. Nurses must also exercise caution to avoid carrying away the client problems or suffering.

Guidelines for Presencing

Your client has just died, and his mother is sobbing at his bedside. Or perhaps you find your client with facial burns in tears after being told she will be permanently disfigured. "What should I say? What is the right thing to do?" the nurse often wonders in such situations. Although presencing is often the most helpful approach to ease suffering, it can at times be difficult to practice. Suggestions for how to practice presencing follow.

Presencing is especially beneficial during times when clients are vulnerable, helpless, or powerless (Pettigrew, 1990). Presencing is effective not only for clients who are dying or in severe physical pain, but also for those who are experiencing spiritual or emotional discomfort. Client vulnerability often reminds nurses of their own vulnerability or woundedness (see Chapter 3). Through the process of self-assessment, nurses can gain insight into their own sense of vulnerability. A nurse might ask: What patient care scenarios make me want to run away? How do I respond to clients with unfixable problems? Do I avoid them? Do I protect myself behind a shield of professionalism?

Nurses under time constraints can find it a challenge to wholeheartedly be present for a client, even for a moment. Snyder, Brandt, and Tseng (2000) suggest that nurses prepare to practice presencing this way: Just before entering a patient room or conducting a home visit, take a moment to focus on the client. Say the client's name, focus attention, and eliminate distractions (Snyder, Brandt, & Tseng). Take several deep, slow breaths while centering. Think the client's name with each inhalation. With each exhalation, think "May I help you [name of patient]?"

When approaching the client, make eye contact and touch the client as is culturally appropriate (Snyder, Brandt, & Tseng, 2000). A verbal exchange may be appropriate, but often during times of deep emotions, spoken language is superficial and superfluous. Silence may be more effective. Presencing is a practice that relies heavily on the nurse's instinct and intuition. To know if, when, and how to touch or to speak should reflect the uniqueness of the situation and the nurse–client relationship. Asking "How would I want someone to be present to me?" can be a good guide for determining how long to maintain eye contact, how to touch, how long to be present, and so forth. A nurse who is invited by the client and able to be sincerely physically, mentally, emotionally, and spiritually present will be able to provide a comforting presence.

A nurse can obtain permission to provide presencing by gently asking the client a simple question like "Would you like to have me be with you awhile?" If, however, asking for permission verbally seems inappropriate, nonverbal permission can be noted by watching a client's body language and evaluating the client's previous behavior in your presence. Does the client appear more relaxed when you are present? Does the client reposition in bed to face you—or to turn away from you? Does the client cling to your hand, or feign sleepiness when you linger?

Bunkers (1999) suggested that eliminating expectations is essential to true presence. Learning to be still, remain open, hear the unspeakable, and witness another's experience of past, present, and future in the current moment are all aspects of presencing. While being present for a client, do not expect anything from the client other than the honor of being present. Presencing does not involve reciprocity; it is a gift to give without "strings attached." The success of presencing should not be measured by client responses (Minicucci, 1998). If a client does not respond with a smile, a "thank you," or a touch, a nurse's presencing can still affect the client powerfully.

Although presencing requires giving of self, the nurse should strive to be a care*giver* and not a care*taker*. Montgomery's (1992) interviews with nurses about their perceptions of caring revealed their wisdom about how to be deeply involved with clients without becoming harmfully overinvolved. The key for these nurses was a "spiritual transcendence" or the ability to see themselves as connected to a greater power. Montgomery observed that this spiritual transcendence was integral to caring and connecting in appropriate and healthful ways, and also provided the energy for caring. Other methods for avoiding overinvolvement include meeting with a counselor who can provide guidance about boundaries with clients or discussing the issue with wise colleagues.

NURSING IMPLICATIONS

The ability to communicate authentically and compassionately is essential to providing care that supports spiritual health. Presencing, a foundational intervention for nurturing the spirit and creating a healing relationship, uses communication skills to convey caring at a deeper level. The research and literature about communication and presencing referred to above suggest a number of implications for nursing practice.

Communicating Presence

Nurses are always communicating, and they are often in the presence of clients. There are various degrees, however, to which the nurse communicates empathy and presence. Although the nurse has the power to determine the level of communication and presencing to employ with a client, choosing to listen holistically and be fully present constitutes effective provision of care and promotes client spiritual healing and health.

Minicucci (1998) suggested that "to the extent that nurses can bring the fullness of their personhood to any patient interaction, the healing resources of the patient are likely to be stimulated" (p. 10). Karl (1992) reflected that the capacity to be present for another is directly related to how well one is connected with that which enlivens. Karl advocated that nurses must be present for themselves first before attempting to be present for others. Answering "Do I live/work/play in ways that bring out the best in me?" and other self-assessment questions (see Chapter 3) can help a nurse prepare to practice presencing.

Effects of a Caring Attitude

The nurse's attitude toward the client is paramount to whether communication or presencing is effective and healing. Evidence suggests that a caring attitude is requisite to effective presencing, caring touch, and empathic listening (Pettigrew, 1990; Rybarczyk & Bellg, 1997; Weiss, 1986). A client will not perceive a nurse's attempts to touch and listen as caring if that nurse does not inwardly maintain a caring attitude toward the client. Nursing knowledge, skill, and experience are ineffectual if not accompanied by caring attitude. Box 4-3 contrasts supportive attitudes of caring with those that are obstructive. Caring attitudes involve compassion, nonjudgmental affirmation, and humility toward clients. Rybarczyk and Bellg suggested that the client's past be honored; that is, the nurse should maintain a sense of wonder and appreciation for the client's story.

Box 4-3. Attitudes that Support/Obstruct Communication

Supportive Attitude	Obstructive Attitude
As much as I am able, I am willing to help you develop healthful responses to your challenges.	I need to fix your problems.
I respect your feelings and thoughts.	I know what you should be feeling (or thinking).
I am willing to be present as you go through your suffering.	The best way to deal with suffering is to avoid or deny it.
Please help me to understand how I may best help you.	I am the professional. I know what is best for you.
I am eager to care for you, even if your behavior annoys/angers/disgusts me.	I am annoyed/angered/disgusted by you.
There is a power greater than ourselves that does the healing/saving.	I do the healing/saving.

Time Constraints

A barrier to empathic listening and presencing among nurses is their perception that they do not have enough time. Listening to distress, especially spiritual distress, is often misperceived as requiring more time than most nurses have for such matters. In an editorial, Meserve (1993) argued that whether or not a client is given focused attention, it takes the same amount of time to be with clients. Meserve contended that intentional noninvolvement on the part of the clinician may actually create more stress than open-hearted concern for clients. Meserve concluded that health care professionals should respect client desires for closeness with them and use that longing to create intimacy for healing purposes. Future research might examine if fulfilling a client's need for an empathic presence and listening could actually save nursing time. Clinical experience shows that a skilled empathic listener can "cut to the chase" and bring about a positive outcome rapidly. Although effective empathic listening requires intense, focused energy, it does not necessarily require excessive amounts of time as Box 4-4 illustrates.

An image that presencing may conjure is one of sitting at a client's bedside for a lengthy period. Nurses rarely have such time to offer. Presencing, however, does not require spending lots of time. "Full" or "transcendent" presencing (Osterman & Schwartz-Barcott, 1996) can be practiced during short intervals while giving a massage or waiting for a topical solution to dry. It may be as brief as the time it takes to give a "knowing look."

Box 4-4. Contrasting Levels of Empathy

Jim, a 23-year-old in the final stages of acute leukemia, is being cared for at home by his mother, Karen. After a home visit, Nurse Lee converses with Karen on the way to her car.

Consider how empathic listening and effective presencing are—or are not—demonstrated in each of the following exchanges:

Exchange A

Karen (mom): Thanks so much for coming.

Lee: Sure . . . no problem.

Karen: It's just so terrible to watch. . . . [voice trails off; eyes tear up]

Lee: I know. At least he isn't in a lot of pain.

Box 4-4. Contrasting Levels of Empathy

Karen: Yeah, I guess that's good. . . . [awkward silence]

Lee: Well, hopefully he'll rest easy tonight.

Karen: Do you mind if I ask you a question?

Lee: Sure, go ahead.

Karen: [long pause] How do you deal with it? I mean its just so unfair, so tragic . . . so [gropes for words]

Lee: Oh, I try to look for the silver lining at times like this. I count my blessings and try to remember the good things in life. And I work hard to manage pain and the other distressing symptoms.

Karen: Oh. Hmmm. Well, I try to care for Jim as best as I can. But that still doesn't. . . .

Lee: Honey, you are such a fabulous mom. And a great nurse too! Jim is lucky to have you. Really.

Karen: [weakly; forces a smile] Well, thanks. I guess you're busy and need to get going. I'll see you next time.

Exchange B

Karen: Thanks so much for coming.

Lee: It's my privilege, Karen.

Karen: It's just so terrible to watch. . . .

Lee: [respectful silence; physical indication of listening]

Karen: How do you deal with it? I mean it's just so unfair, so tragic. . . .

Lee: It is unfair for someone to suffer and die prematurely. Such suffering often raises lots of questions and issues. [thoughtful silence] How are you dealing with it?

Karen: [begins to sob] It's overwhelming. But I think the worst part is that it is shaking my beliefs. I mean why would a loving God do this to my son? To me? I try to pray and it just doesn't seem to work.

Lee: [comfortable silence] I hear your anguish, Karen. I find myself feeling some of it. I'm not able to give the perfect answer, but I am wanting to be with you while you struggle with the questions [hugs; tears up].

KEY POINTS

- Empathic listening and presencing are skills requisite to spiritual caregiving and serve as cornerstones for other spiritual care strategies.
- Empathic listening can occur at different levels. The most therapeutic is holistic listening, which involves a listener's attending to the intellectual, emotional, physical, and spiritual content of the client message.
- Procedural and nonprocedural caring touch can create positive client outcomes when the nurse maintains an attitude of caring.
- Presencing involves giving of self and being available to clients and attentive in a way that is meaningful for them.
- Critical elements of presencing include vulnerability, silence, invitation, and privilege (Pettigrew, 1990).
- Nurses have identified different levels of presencing. The most advanced level of presencing occurs when a nurse is physically, mentally, emotionally, and spiritually present for a client.
- Nurses recognize many positive outcomes of presencing, including diminished suffering and decreased anxiety and sense of isolation.
- Nursing strategies for effective presencing include:
  - Being aware of ways they may attempt to avoid spiritual pain and suffering in order to overcome such avoidance when they observe their clients experiencing spiritual discomfort
  - Centering before entering into the presence of clients
  - Using eye contact and touch appropriately
  - Gaining permission from the client to be present
  - Limiting expectations of the client
  - Recognizing that presencing does not require long periods of time with a client (even a knowing look can be helpful)
  - Avoiding overinvolvement by maintaining appropriate boundaries.

LOOK WITHIN TO LEARN

1. Recall the last time you felt that someone really comforted you. What was it about the presence of this person that was comforting? What did this person do that made you feel understood, secure, or cared for?

2. How do you typically respond when a client (or other person) begins to cry? Do you think your response is helpful? How would you want a nurse to respond to you if you were crying?

3. Imagine that you are working on a busy unit with a heavy caseload. One of your clients appears to be very frightened and seems to need to talk. You think, "But I don't have time!" What strategies might you implement to address your client's needs?

4. To the best of your ability, write down verbatim a recent conversation with another person you were trying to help. Ask yourself: In what ways did I communicate caring? What level of empathy did I display? Did I in any way avoid or devalue the person's problem or pain?

5. Montgomery (1992) and McKivergin (2000) suggest that nurses can remain effective, healing presences for clients by being conduits for a spiritual energy that emanates from a transcendent source (e.g., God). Do you agree? Why or why not?

REFERENCES

Bold print indicates those that are most recommended.

Balzer-Riley, J. W. (1996). *Communication in nursing* (3rd ed.). St. Louis, MO: Mosby.

Bunkers, S. S. (1999). Learning to be still. *Nursing Science Quarterly, 12*(2), 172–173.

Emblen, J. D., & Halstead, L. (1993). Spiritual needs and interventions: Comparing the views of patients, nurses, and chaplains. *Clinical Nurse Specialist, 1,* 175–182.

Estabrooks, C. A., & Morse, J. M. (1992). Toward a theory of touch: The touching process and acquiring a touching style. *Journal of Advanced Nursing, 17,* 448–456.

Fortinash, K. M., & Holoday-Worret, P. A. (Eds.). (2000). *Psychiatric mental health nursing* (2nd ed.). St. Louis, MO: Mosby.

Fredriksson, L. (1999). Modes of relating in a caring conversation: A research synthesis on presence, touch, and listening. *Journal of Advanced Nursing, 30,* 1167–1176.

Gardner, D. (1992). Presence. In G. Bulechek & J. McCloskey (Eds.), *Nursing interventions: Treatments for nursing diagnoses* (2nd ed., pp. 316–324). Philadelphia: Saunders.

Hauerwas, S. (1990). *Naming the silences: God, medicine, and the problem of suffering.* Grand Rapids, MI: Eerdmans.

Karl, J. C. (1992). Being there: Who do you bring to practice? In D. A. Gaut (Ed.), *The presence of caring in nursing* (pp. 1–13). New York: National League for Nursing [Publ. No. 15-2465].

McKivergin, M. (2000). The nurse as an instrument of healing. In B. M. Dassey, L. Keegan, & C. E. Guzzetta (Eds.), *Holistic nursing: A handbook for practice* (3rd ed.) (pp. 207–227). Gaithersburg, MD: Aspen.

Meserve, H. C. (1993). Editorial. *Journal of Religion and Health, 32*(2), 89–90.

Minicucci, D. S. (1998). A review and synthesis of the literature: The use of presence in the nursing care of families. *Journal of the New York State Nurses Association, 29*(3/4), 9–15.

Montgomery, C. L. (1992). The spiritual connection: Nurses' perceptions of the experience of caring. In D. A. Gaut (Ed.), *The presence of caring in nursing.* (pp. 9–52). New York: National League for Nursing [Publ. No. 15-2465].

Myers, S. (2000). Empathic listening: Reports on the experience of being heard. *Journal of Humanistic Psychology, 40,* 148–173.

Oglesby, W. B., Jr. (1980). *Biblical themes for pastoral care.* Nashville: Abington.

Osterman, P., & Schwartz-Barcott, D. (1996). Presence: Four ways of being there. *Nursing Forum, 31*(2), 23–30.

Pettigrew, J. (1990). Intensive nursing care: The ministry of presence. *Critical Care Nursing Clinics of North America, 2,* 503–508.

Rowan, J. (1986). Holistic listening. *Journal of Humanistic Psychology, 26*(1), 83–102.

Rybarczyk, B., & Bellg, A. (1997). *Listening to life stories.* New York: Springer.

Sellers, S. C., & Haag, B. A. (1998). Spiritual nursing interventions. *Journal of Holistic Nursing, 16,* 338–354.

Snyder, M., Brandt, C. L., & Tseng, Y. (2000). Use of presence in the critical care unit. *AACN Clinical issues: Advanced Practice in Acute & Critical Care, 11*(1), 27–33.

Taylor, E. J., Amenta, M. O., & Highfield, M. F. (1995). Spiritual care practices of oncology nurses. *Oncology Nursing Forum, 22*(1), 31–39.

Weiss, S. J. (1986). Psychophysiologic effects of caregiver touch on incidence of cardiac dysrhythmia. *Heart & Lung, 15,* 495–505.

Zerwekh, J. V. (1997). The practice of presencing. *Seminars in Oncology Nursing, 13,* 260–262.

5

Spiritual Assessment

When we consider aspects of a client's health, whether physiologic, psychosocial, or spiritual, or all of these dimensions, assessment is the first step. Before taking action to treat a pressure sore, for example, the nurse must verify the presence of a pressure sore, determine its size and characteristics, and identify factors that may mediate treatments and their outcomes. Without the information a careful and thorough assessment provides, effective treatment is compromised. So it is with spiritual caregiving.

Before planning care for spiritual needs, the nurse must conduct an adequate assessment. Working with the client, the nurse seeks to discover:

nurse discovers

- Does the client have spiritual needs?
- What is the nature of these needs?
- What factors contribute to these needs?
- How do certain beliefs, experiences, relationships, or the current illness influence these needs?
- What does the client think might help to address these needs?
- Does the client want help?
- From whom will the client accept help?

Identifying religious affiliation or determining if a client wishes to see a chaplain is often the extent of a spiritual assessment in many health care institutions. Such a limited focus does not provide adequate understanding of a client's spiritual needs. Signs of spiritual needs may be confused with indicators of what are primarily psychosocial needs (Highfield & Cason, 1983). Yet a nurse with some sensitivity and guidance can complete a basic spiritual assessment.

purpose   The purpose of this chapter is to guide nurses to conduct spiritual assessments. After reviewing selected models for spiritual assessment and relevant nursing research, the chapter offers practical suggestions to facilitate assessment of spiritual needs. Barriers to conducting spiritual assessment and strategies for overcoming them will also be presented.

MODELS FOR SPIRITUAL ASSESSMENT

A number of nurse authors (Carpenito, 1995; Dossey, 1998; Highfield, 1993, 1997; Highfield & Cason, 1983; O'Brien, 1999; Peterson, 1987; Stoll, 1979; Yeadon, 1986) offer guidance about spiritual assessment. Much wisdom about the topic stems also from the fields of pastoral care and chaplaincy, psychiatry, and psychology (Fitchett, 1993; Maloney, 1993; Muncy, 1996; Pruyser, 1976; VandeCreek, Ayres, & Bassham, 1995; van der Poel, 1998); these disciplines have influenced how nurses think about spiritual assessment. A few physicians have also published descriptions of approaches to spiritual assessment (Koenig & Pritchett, 1998; Maugens, 1996; Salisbury, Ciulla, & McSherry, 1989). Most of these authors offer a model for spiritual assessment that incorporates a list of categories or dimensions of spirituality. These models are helpful, because they suggest what to include in a thorough spiritual assessment. Although they have not been tested by clinical research, the following selected models are supported by valid scholarly inquiry and clinical experience. As with other aspects of spiritual care, spiritual assessment is an important new area for research.

Nursing Models

In a classic article, Stoll (1979) identified that a comprehensive spiritual assessment involves asking clients questions that tap each of four dimensions. Stoll's four areas for spiritual assessment include:

- The client's concept of God or deity (e.g., What are your beliefs about God or a higher power? How do these beliefs help you during difficult times?)
- Sources of hope and strength (e.g., What gives you courage while you are sick?)
- Religious practices (e.g., What religious habits or rituals comfort you when you are discouraged?)
- The relationship between spiritual beliefs and health (e.g., How does your spirituality affect the way you live with your health challenges?)

Stoll implies that spiritual assessment can be a one-time event, an intake assessment that guides care throughout the remainder of the client's admission.

In the 1980s, Highfield (1983) introduced pastoral counselor Clinebell's categories of spiritual need into nursing. Highfield identified client behaviors and statements that may indicate spiritual needs. Highfield's work suggested the prevalence of spiritual needs and the frequency with which they are expressed without the use of religious language. These categories include:

- The need to give love (e.g., feeling a burden to others because illness prevents reciprocating loving care)
- The need to receive love (e.g., feeling alone or abandoned)
- The need for hope and creativity (e.g., feeling despair or being bored while ill)
- The need for meaning and purpose (e.g., wondering "why?")

Later, Highfield (1993) introduced the PLAN model for spiritual assessment and care, an approach that encourages nurses to practice in a manner that reflects their own abilities and limitations, as well as the unique concerns of the client. The PLAN model follows four increasingly complex tiers: **P**ermission, **L**imited information, **A**ctivating resources, and **N**on-nursing referrals. The first level involves gaining permission by encouraging the client to understand that it is appropriate to discuss spiritual concerns with a nurse. Next, the nurse provides limited information in response to concerns raised by the client. The third and fourth tiers of Highfield's PLAN model involve activating resources (based on a more in-depth spiritual assessment) to assist the client toward spiritual well-being, and making non-nursing referrals when the nurse is not equipped to address the client's spiritual concerns.

Carpenito's (2000) questions for collecting data to formulate a nursing diagnoses of "spiritual distress" or "potential for enhanced spiritual well-being" reflect Stoll's (1979) and Highfield's (1983) approaches. Carpenito suggested that nurses assess for defining characteristics of spiritual distress by asking questions that ascertain a client's source of spiritual strength and meaning, spiritual practices, presence of a spiritual leader, and how spiritual beliefs affect health. Carpenito also recommends that nurses ask clients how they can assist them to maintain their spiritual strength. Objective data for formulating a diagnosis of spiritual distress can be found by noting client involvement in spiritual activities and practices, as well as client response to the spiritual assessment interview. Carpenito proposes that subjective data supporting the diagnosis of Potential for Enhanced Spiritual Well-Being can be elicited from client comments about a "trust relationship with or in the transcendent," meaning and hope, and inner strength and peace.

Dossey (1998) offered a spiritual assessment tool with language that is less traditional (i.e., less overtly religious). This tool includes questions designed to assess the following aspects of spirituality:

- **Meaning and purpose:** The ability to seek meaning and fulfillment in life, manifest hope, and accept ambiguity and uncertainty
- **Inner strength:** The ability to manifest joy and recognize strengths, choices, goals, and faith
- **Interconnections:** positive self-concept, self-esteem, and sense of self; sense of belonging in the world with others; capacity to pursue personal interests; and ability to demonstrate love of self and self-forgiveness

Thus far, Dossey's assessment tool is the most comprehensive in the nursing literature; its categories reflect the breadth of spirituality identified by nurses over the past 20 to 30 years.

Other Models

Models for assessing the spiritual dimension have long existed outside of the discipline of nursing. Some of these models provide new insight regarding categories for which to assess, and others contribute strategies for conducting a comprehensive assessment.

Pruyser (1976) proposed seven dimensions or traits of spirituality. Each dimension can be considered a continuum with negative and unhealthy versus positive and healthy parameters. For example, a client with a healthy sense of the sacred (or "awareness of the holy") may be heard to exclaim, "I feel very spiritual now . . . that Someone is with me," whereas a client with a weaker sense of the holy might say, "If there is a God, He isn't interested in me." Box 5-1 summarizes Pruyser's dimensions and exemplifies each end of the continuum with statements that clients or their loved ones might make.

Box 5-1. Pruyser's Spiritual Dimensions as Interpreted by Maloney (1993) and Kloss (1988)

Box 5-1. Pruyser's Seven Dimensions of Spirituality		
Dimension	**Continuum**	
	Positive/Healthy	**Negative/Unhealthy**
1. Awareness of the Holy or God (how much an individual senses awe, reverence for that which is divine)	"I feel very close to God now and am dependent on God's help to get well again."	"When I hear the birds sing, they mock me; I see nothing sacred in nature—or anything else."
2. Acceptance of God's grace and steadfast love (how much one experiences God as benevolent and unconditional in loving)	"Thank you for caring for me so tenderly; you mirror God for me."	"I don't need or deserve any help or kindness; I'll handle things alone."

(continues)

Box 5-1. Pruyser's Spiritual Dimensions as Interpreted by Maloney (1993) and Kloss (1988) *(continued)*

Box 5-1. Pruyser's Seven Dimensions of Spirituality		
Dimension	**Continuum**	
	Positive/Healthy	**Negative/Unhealthy**
3. Faith (how much one is open, committed, and positive about life)	"I've enjoyed every minute of life! I try anything new."	"There are many things in life I'd be afraid to do."
4. Being repentant and responsible (how much one is open to change and responsible for his or her own feelings and behaviors)	"How can I deal with my situation better?"	"It's not my fault I feel bitter."
5. Sense of providence (how much one experiences God's leadership and direction)	"I trust that God's will will be done in my life and illness."	"Where has God been for me? He left me when I got sick."
6. Involvement in spiritual/religious community, and experience of communion	"I still feel connected to my church because I know that they are praying for me."	"Why should I have to ask for help from my church? They don't bother to even call me!"
7. Flexibility and commitment to living an ethical life	"Even though I'm sick, I think my life is sacred; I still have much to offer the world."	"There is no reason for me to still live; just let me die."

Maloney

Maloney (1993) asserted that Pruyser's seven dimensions required an additional dimension and labeled this trait as "openness in faith." Maloney believed that openness in faith prevents individual rigidity or resistance to new ideas in spiritual beliefs. Although, as Pruyser and Maloney acknowledge, this model is molded by Christian perspectives, it offers insight into spiritual dimensions or categories that may manifest among non-Christians and thus has application for them as well.

Muncy

Muncy (1996) fused aspects of spirituality and suggested assessing three dimensions. First, Muncy recommends exploring client self-understanding and attitudes about others. Muncy posits that how clients view themselves and others frequently reveals their view of God. For example, individuals who have difficulty forgiving themselves or others may be more likely to view God as unforgiving. Second, Muncy suggests assessing religious and spiritual history, including sense of purpose. Knowledge of a client's spiritual background and purpose in life helps a nurse to understand factors that influence a client's experience of illness or other health challenges. Finally, and what is unique from other models presented, Muncy advocates asking clients about their spiritual goals, which creates an opportunity for the clinician to discuss with the client a plan for spiritual care.

Maugens

Although it does not introduce a new category for spiritual assessment, a device offered by Maugens (1996) assists nurses in remembering components to cover during a spiritual assessment. Maugens's mnemonic SPIRIT for spiritual history is:

- "Spiritual belief system" refers to religious affiliation and theology. Knowledge about client beliefs assists the nurse to make appropriate referrals if necessary, and to understand how these beliefs affect response to illness or decisions about treatment.
- "Personal spirituality" refers to the spiritual views that are shaped by life experiences, unique to the individual, and not necessarily related to religious belief. A client, for example, may have experienced a spiritual transformation after a near-death experience and not necessarily consider it a religious experience.
- "Integration and involvement with a spiritual community" indicates a client's membership and role in a religious organization or other group that provides spiritual support. Knowledge that a spiritual community supports a client allows a nurse to discuss with the client how this community's spiritual resources can be utilized, and if appropriate, to incorporate this community in the client's care. The

nurse also discusses with the client how to remain active in the community despite illness imposed confinement.

- "**R**itualized practices and restrictions" are behaviors and lifestyle activities that influence health. These include diet, worship practices, prayer rituals, or holy days that may influence the needs of a client coping with health challenges.
- "**I**mplications" for health care as part of the SPIRITual history reminds the nurse to assess how spiritual beliefs and practices influence the client's desire and participation in health care. For example, the knowledge that a client believes cure comes only from God rather than the assistance of health care professionals provides the nurse insight about how to discuss treatment options.
- "**T**erminal events planning" reminds the clinician to assess end-of-life concerns. This aspect of the SPIRITual history is especially appropriate for terminally ill clients, but sometimes warranted for others. The nurse who assesses beliefs about an afterlife, cremation, meaning of death, and so forth, can provide more sensitive care for clients for whom death is imminent.

Fitchett (1993) developed a model for spiritual assessment that encompasses seven dimensions. These include:

1. Beliefs and meaning (i.e., mission, purpose, religious and nonreligious meaning in life)
2. Authority and guidance (i.e., exploring where or with whom one places trusts, seeks guidance)
3. Experience (i.e., of the divine or demonic) and emotion (i.e., the tone emerging from one's spiritual experience)
4. Fellowship (i.e., involvement in any formal or informal community that shares spiritual beliefs and practices)
5. Ritual and practice (i.e., activities that make life meaningful)
6. Courage and growth (i.e., the ability to encounter doubt and inner change)
7. Vocation and consequences (i.e., what persons believe they should do, what is their calling)

A case study (Box 5-2) illustrates how this model is applied to a client interview.

Salisbury, Ciulla, and McSherry (1989) proposed four major areas for spiritual assessment. These areas include assessment of the significant others of the client (e.g., who influences their sense of love, connected-

---

Box 5-2. Applying Fitchett's (1993) Model: One Nurse's Story

Lynne, a 43-year-old Roman Catholic woman living with recurrent breast cancer metastasized to the spine, is married, has an 11-year-old son, and lives in an upper-middle-class suburb. Lynne was receiving chemotherapy at a major university hospital. Excerpts from a home interview provide a partial picture of Lynne's spirituality. Although other models for spiritual assessment could be applied, Fitchett's was selected because of its comprehensiveness.

Lynne: When I was feeling well, I was active and able to maintain my good spirits. Now I go to the Wellness Center every week. And even though I had a pounding headache and had to drag myself there this week, I was determined to go. I get a lot from going, so I went. I felt like doodoo, but I went! [laughs] Yeah, my emotional state is really tied into my physical state. I've been thinking that I've got to do something about that. It might be something I want to talk to my support group friends about. The feeling that I am in a body that is unsafe. Safety has to come from someplace else now rather than from controlling every single thing, including my body.

Nurse: So where does this safety come from?

Lynne: I'm not sure yet. That's why I go to the Wellness Center. I think it has something to do with spirituality. And I'm not a real religious person, but it has something to do with me that's not physical. . . . I haven't done art work in years. And I thought, well maybe that's something I can do. So far, I can still use my hands, so I don't have to lift, push, pull, or bend. So a friend bought me a big hunk of clay, and I'm thinking I'll do some sculpture. And at least it'll be something. I feel like I'm not productive. I don't know why I feel I have to be productive every minute! That's part of my old neurosis. . . .

I have always been involved in work that involved other people's tragedies. I was a patient consultant at the local hospital for five years. So I had to deal with people who had cancer or heart problems, parents of children with congenital defects. I worked with inner city youth, who had lots of problems—as you can well imagine! And so, I thought I was a great problem solver, but I never had to solve problems for myself, because I was never challenged. But I don't know . . . what's to solve here? It's all that inner, spiritual stuff. It gets back to that. So I don't know.

(continues)

Box 5-2. Applying Fitchett's (1993) Model: One Nurse's Story (continued)

All the things I want to be involved in with my son. [cries] Taking him to school. Being able to give him advice. He'll have a dad, a grandmother . . . but he won't have me. And then, part of me says that's really arrogant.

Trying to search for meaning and why you have cancer is a lot like chasing your tail. [voice cracks] I alternate between thinking its a crapshoot—a celestial crapshoot, perhaps, but a crapshoot nonetheless. That it could be the lady across the street as well as me. And then other times I think there has to be a reason for this. [voice even more unsteady now] I wish I could figure out what it is. I know I am more able to let people do things for me. And maybe that's what I need to learn in life [cries]. . . .

Analysis

Belief and Meaning: Lynne explicitly describes her distress caused by questions of meaning, the meaning of her illness, her life, and her eventual death. She is struggling to determine if she is a victim of a "celestial crapshoot" or a purposeful, ordered universe.

Authority and Guidance: Prior to her illness, Lynne saw herself as being able to answer the questions of life satisfactorily; now authority of self is challenged. She wonders where to turn for comfort, security, direction, and answers. During the interview, she mentioned that since her diagnosis, she has begun to pray to her grandmother, whom she saw as a saint. She does find guidance from her support group, relaxation tapes, and books on coping with cancer.

Experience and Emotion: Lynne's spiritual issues manifest in anxiety, anger, and sorrow. Amidst Lynne's distress, there is an appreciation for the self-insight she has gained from her cancer experience. She also recognizes a direct relationship between how she feels physically and her "spirits."

Fellowship: Lynne's precancer involvement in her community, which gave her a great sense of purpose, has been curtailed because of her cancer. However, she does thrive on her relationships with her husband, son, and friends who have remained loyal.

Ritual and Practice: Presently, most religious practices fail to bring

Box 5-2. Applying Fitchett's (1993) Model: One Nurse's Story *(concluded)*

comfort to Lynne. Her art work, however, will allow her to pray, to express herself in a meaningful way. Her art work is also a way for her to leave a legacy, another way to create a sense of meaning for her life.

Courage and Growth: Lynne's courage is exhibited by her ability to enter spiritual doubt, to face the "dark night of the soul." Although she is not satisfied with the answers (or lack thereof) to her many spiritual questions, she is allowing for spiritual maturation by entering into struggle. It is struggle and doubt that precedes breakthrough, turn-arounds, learning, and growth.

Vocation: What duties and obligations make Lynne's life purposeful? Lynne finds meaning in being a mother, wife, and friend and in creating beauty and joy for others through her art work.

ness, and community?), the quality of relationship with God and religion, spiritual resources, and spiritual concerns. These clinicians developed a checklist form for documenting client responses to spiritual assessment questions. The form lists specific spiritual concerns that are common among hospitalized patients. These include:

- Anger toward God
- Grief and anticipatory grief
- Concerns about dying and afterlife
- Inner conflict about beliefs
- Shame
- Unrelieved guilt
- Questions about why God coexists with evil and suffering
- Concerns related to the moral or ethical nature of medical treatments

Salisbury, Ciulla, and McSherry's contribution to spiritual assessment practice is the systematization of documentation about client spirituality. A concrete codification of spiritual concerns allows clinicians and researchers to communicate easily about a client's spirituality, and allows client spiritual concerns to be compared and statistically analyzed with other quantifiable factors.

Summary of Spiritual Assessment Models

The spiritual assessment models reviewed propose specific aspects of spirituality for which to assess. Most of these models identify dimensions of spirituality that overlap with other models, perhaps with different labeling. Some of the models are helpful not because they introduce new dimensions for which to assess, but because of the strategies they suggest will aid assessment (e.g., Maugens, 1996). A summary of these models is found in Box 5-3.

Box 5-3. Spiritual Assessment Models Summarized		
Author/ Discipline	**Dimensions of Spirituality**	**Unique Contribution**
Stoll/Nursing *see p. 105*	(a) Concept of deity or God (b) Sources of strength and hope (c) Religious practices (d) Relationship between spiritual beliefs and health	First widely disseminated model used by nurses
Highfield/ Nursing *see p. 105*	(a) Need to give love (b) Need to receive love (c) Need for hope and creativity (d) Need for meaning and purpose	Introduced a chaplain's model to nurses; illustrated concepts with observable indicators

Box 5-3. Spiritual Assessment Models Summarized *(continued)*		
Author/ Discipline	**Dimensions of Spirituality**	**Unique Contribution**
Carpenito/ Nursing *see p. 106*	(a) Subjective data—defining characteristics: spiritual practices, sources of strength and meaning, presence of a spiritual leader, affect of health challenge on beliefs; related factors—how nurse can assist to maintain spiritual strength (b) Objective data—current practices, response to spiritual assessment, participation in spiritual practices	Offered as requisite to a diagnosis of spiritual distress
Dossey/ Nursing *see p. 106 & p. 119*	(a) Meaning and purpose (b) Inner strength (c) Interconnections	Avoids religious biases in use of language; offers specific assessment questions for clinical use
Pruyser/ Psychology and Pastoral Counseling *see p. 107-8*	(a) Awareness of holy, God (b) Acceptance of grace and love (c) Faith and commitment to life (d) Repentance and responsibility (e) Sense of providence (f) Involvement in spiritual community	Seminal work influencing chaplains for decades; introduced notion that spiritual problems could be "diagnosed"

(continues)

Author/ Discipline	Dimensions of Spirituality	Unique Contribution
Muncy/ Chaplaincy *see p 109*	(a) Self-understanding and attitudes toward others (b) Religious and spiritual history (c) Spiritual goals	Allows for identification of what clients perceive to be their spiritual goals
Maugens/ Medicine *see p 109*	(a) Spiritual beliefs (b) Personal spirituality (c) Integration in a spiritual community (d) Rituals and restrictions (e) Implications for health care (f) Terminal events planning	Offers a mnemonic for remembering assessment components *SPIRIT. takes 10-15 min*
Fitchett/ Chaplaincy *see p.110-3*	(a) Belief and meaning (b) Authority and guidance (c) Experience and emotion (d) Fellowship and community (e) Ritual and practices (f) Courage and growth (g) Vocation	Comprehensive; reflects work of multidisciplinary team
McSherry and colleagues/ Medicine *see p113*	(a) Relations with significant others (b) Relations with God and religion (c) Spiritual resources (d) Spiritual concerns	Moves clinicians toward quantifying and coding spiritual concerns

Box 5-3. Spiritual Assessment Models Summarized *(concluded)*

RESEARCH ON SPIRITUAL ASSESSMENT

Nurse researchers who have empirically studied spiritual assessment have done so to describe its prevalence and process (Boutell & Bozett, 1987; Highfield & Cason, 1983; Highfield, 1991). Highfield observed that oncology nurses often failed to recognize client spiritual needs and mistook spiritual needs for psychosocial needs (Highfield, Highfield & Cason). Boutell and Bozett (1987) surveyed 238 Oklahoma nurses providing direct patient care and found that 34 percent reported assessing spiritual needs often or always and 38 percent reported doing so occasionally. Boutell and Bozett conjectured that this high rate of perceived spiritual assessment may be related to the fact that 74 percent of this sample were actively involved in churches. Social workers Dudley and colleagues' (1995) research involved analyzing the content of spiritual assessment forms returned from 53 hospices. They observed that these forms included questions pertaining to patient religious affiliation, issues, problems or barriers, rituals, and spirituality (unrelated to religion). Forms contained open-ended questions as well as questions related to the plan for spiritual care.

A growing number of researchers have developed and tested research instruments for quantifying clients' spirituality (e.g., Hungelmann, Kenkel-Rossi, Klassen, & Stollenwerk, 1989; O'Brien, 1999; Reed, 1987). Typically, these "paper-and-pencil" instruments allow the respondent to answer two pages or more of questions. These instruments can be time consuming, confusing for poorly educated clients, and culturally insensitive for persons who are not religious or believe in "God." It is theoretically possible that research instruments can be used for clinical purposes to assess client spirituality. Two research teams have proposed that their spirituality instruments are applicable to clinical assessment purposes (O'Brien, 1999; Salisbury, Ciulla, & McSherry, 1989). A research instrument used or adapted for clinical practice, however, does need to be short (perhaps fewer than 10 to 15 items), free of religiously biased language, easily scored or interpreted, and adaptable to various client circumstances. Investigation of the appropriateness, sensitivity, or feasibility of quantitative spiritual assessment tools in clinical practice is an area for future research.

CONDUCTING A SPIRITUAL ASSESSMENT

Because spirituality is an integral and determining force for people—especially when they are facing health challenges—it is important for nurses to know about client spirituality. A client's spiritual history provides the health care team with valuable information about what gives this client a purpose for living, what beliefs influence treatment decisions and compliance, what spiritual pains may be hindering physical health, and so forth. Or, put colloquially, information from a spiritual assessment helps the nurse understand something about what makes clients "tick" and what "boosts their spirits." The models just reviewed can guide nurses in conducting the assessment that is essential to an understanding of a client's unique spiritual status.

The review of spiritual assessment models introduces the reader to the complexity of human spirituality and the commonality of manifestations of spirituality among all people. Until the nurse acquires expertise in conducting spiritual assessments, it may be overwhelming or intimidating to consider conducting such an assessment. However, the nurse who applies the same caution and wisdom necessary for other nursing responsibilities to spiritual assessment will succeed.

Guidelines for Spiritual Assessment

Burkhardt and Nagai-Jacobson (1985) and Highfield (1993) advocate a two-tiered approach to assessment that suggests that nurses pursue an in-depth or focused assessment only after observing indicators of spiritual distress. That is, it is efficient and appropriate for the nurse to first conduct a brief, general assessment of clients' spirituality, then focus subsequent spiritual assessment on specific areas found to be of concern. Following this approach to spiritual assessment makes sense considering time constraints that nurses confront in today's health care environment. An approach that is based on observed indicators of spiritual need also decreases the likelihood of inappropriate meddling. The following procedure can guide nurses.

On admission, the nurse conducts a brief assessment that ascertains the following:

- General spiritual status (e.g., "How are your spirits now?")
- Spiritual needs (e.g., "What kinds of spiritual concerns bother you most?")
- Spiritual resources (e.g., "What do you think might help you with these concerns? In what ways can members of your health care team boost your spirits?")

Either a verbal or written format can be used to conduct this brief assessment. To more completely assess the general spiritual status of a client, a list of questions could address various spiritual dimensions. After this brief assessment, if spiritual concerns are evident, the nurse either plans time for further assessment or makes a referral to a spiritual care specialist.

Focused Spiritual Assessment

The nurse should continue to assess spiritual status, needs, and resources during the period of the nurse–client relationship. When specific spiritual problems are identified during the general assessment, the nurse can conduct a focused spiritual assessment to better understand those specific problems. If a nurse who is guided by Dossey's model observes a sense of dis-ease or need in a client with regard to having meaning and purpose, inner strength, or maintaining interconnectedness (with self, others, or a transcendent other), this nurse will probe further to assess what the problem is definitively and what can be done to help. For example, if a client indicates he is having difficulty with the spiritual resource of prayer, assess further what the difficulty is, what help is wanted, what the difficulty with praying means, and so forth. This focused assessment could include questions like the following:

- You mentioned that you have been having difficulty praying since you were diagnosed; can you tell me more about what you think is creating this challenge for you? Is it related to the emotional stress of your illness, or to the medications, or something else?
- How does not being able to pray affect you?
- In what ways might we be able to assist you in resuming or understanding healing prayer practices?

For another example, if a nurse observes a terminally ill client's spouse crying and stating, "Why does God have to take my sweetheart?", then the nurse would want to understand further what factors may contribute to or relieve this spiritual pain. To focus the assessment on the pertinent topic, the nurse would then ask questions that explore the spouse's "why?" questions, beliefs about misfortune, perceptions of God, and spiritual coping strategies.

If assessing a complex spiritual problem that requires more expertise, the nurse consults a spiritual care specialist (e.g., trained chaplain). See Chapter 8 for more information about making a referral.

Assessment Strategies

Timing

It is common practice in health care organizations to assess religious affiliation upon admission. Most hospices routinely complete a spiritual assessment at admission (Dudley, Smith, & Millison, 1995). However, some experts maintain that spiritual assessment should be an ongoing endeavor (Maugens, 1996; Peterson, 1987). Generally, nurses are not assessing adequately when they ask one or two questions about religion or spirituality during an intake interview. As detailed above, spiritual assessment should be ongoing throughout the nurse–client relationship. Stoll (1979) recognized the significance of timing when asking clients questions about spirituality. Stoll suggested that spiritual assessment be separated from an assessment of sexuality, because both topics are sensitive and intimate.

Establishing Rapport and Trust

Because clients will have difficulty discussing the intimate topic of spirituality with a nurse whom they do not trust, it is essential for the nurse to establish rapport (McSherry, 1996; Peterson, 1987; Stoll, 1979). Rapport can be established more quickly when a nurse consistently demonstrates an attitude of respect and compassion towards the client. In contrast, the nurse who has become desensitized to suffering, is "burned out," or projects personal discomfort with spiritual matters will likely have difficulty establishing rapport with clients. In addition to maintaining authenticity and empathy, the nurse can utilize basic communication strategies presented in Chapter 4 to establish rapport and trust with a client.

Because spirituality and religiosity are personal topics (as are many topics nurses assess), it is polite for a nurse to preface a spiritual assessment by acknowledging the sensitivity of this dimension (Maugens, 1996; Stoll, 1979; Taylor, 2001). Such a preface can also be a way of seeking permission, the first step in conducting an assessment according to Highfield's PLAN model (1993). Maugens suggested this approach to introducing the spiritual assessment:

> Many people have strong spiritual or religious beliefs that shape their lives, including their health and experiences with illness. If you are comfortable talking about this topic, would you please share any of your beliefs and practices that you might want me to know. . . . (p. 12)

Other approaches could include:

> There is recent research that supports a connection between our physical and spiritual health. To help us know more about what influences your overall health, I would like to ask you some questions about your spirituality.

As a nurse, I am eager to care for you as a whole person—physically, psychosocially, and spiritually. So I would like to know more about the spiritual part of you.

Introductions such as these will likely help both the client and the clinician to feel at ease during the assessment.

Appropriate Language

Because asking a client questions is an integral part of most spiritual assessments, it is good to remember some of the basics of formulating good questions. Asking close-ended questions that allow for short, factual or yes/no responses is helpful when a nurse truly has no time or ability for further assessment. Otherwise, to appreciate the uniqueness and complexity of an individual's spirituality, the nurse will do well to focus on asking open-ended questions. The best open-ended questions begin with how, what, when, who, or phrases like "Tell me about. . . ." Generally, questions beginning with why are not helpful; they are often mixed with a sense of threat or challenge (e.g., "Why do you believe that?"). Box 5-4 provides a

---

Box 5-4. Dimensions of Spirituality with Corresponding Assessment Questions

Experience of <u>God or Transcendence</u>

Is religion or God important to you? Why or why not?

Does God/Higher Power/Ultimate Other/The Transcendent/etc. seem personal to you? Do you feel close now?

How does God or a deity function in your personal life?

How is God working in your life?

How would you describe your God and what you worship?

What is your picture of God?

What do you feel you mean to God?

Are there any barriers between you and God? Is there anything you think God could not forgive you?

How do you make sense of feeling angry at God?

How does God respond when you pray?

(continues)

Box 5-4. Dimensions of Spirituality with Corresponding Assessment Questions *(continued)*

Do you feel a source of love from God or any spiritual being?

Where is God in all this?

Spirit-Enhancing Practices or Rituals

How do you express your spirituality (or philosophy of life)?

What spiritual or religious practices or activities that are important to you?

How has being sick affected your spiritual practices?

How does being sick have an impact on your praying (or meditation, scripture reading, fasting, receiving sacraments, service attendance, etc.)?

How and for what do you pray?

What spiritual or religious books or symbols are helpful to you?

What effect do you expect your illness to have on your spiritual practices or beliefs?

What kinds of readings, artwork, or music are inspirational for you?

How do Holy Scriptures (e.g., Koran, Bible) help you in daily life?

How can I as a nurse help you with your spiritual practices?

How do your religious practices help you to grow spiritually?

Involvement in a Spiritual Community (e.g., Church, Temple, Covenant Group)

How involved in a spiritual/religious community/organization are you? (As a visitor? Member? Leader?)

What kind of relationship do you have with the leader of your spiritual community (e.g., priest, rabbi, guru)?

In what ways does your spiritual community help you when times are bad?

What kinds of confusion or doubt do you have about your religious beliefs?

Are you having difficulty carrying out your religious duties?

Box 5-4. Dimensions of Spirituality with Corresponding Assessment Questions *(continued)*

Sense of Meaning

What gives most meaning to your life? What is the most important thing in your life?

When you are sick do you have feelings that you are being punished? Or that it is God's will for you to be sick?

What are your thoughts about or explanations for suffering? Are these beliefs helpful?

What do you see as the cosmic/God's plan or purpose for your life?

Have you been able to answer any of the "why" questions that often accompany illness?

What, if any, have been the good outcomes from having this difficult time in life?

What, if anything, motivates you to get well?

Giving and Receiving Love, or Connectedness to Self (Degree of Self-Awareness) and Others

What do you do to show love for yourself?

What are some of the most loving things that people have done for you? What are the loving things that you do for others?

How do others help you now? How easy is it to accept their help?

For what do you hope? How do you experience hope?

How have you experienced forgiveness during your life/illness? (Forgiveness toward self, toward or from others and God)

Sources of Hope and Strength

What helps you to cope now?

What (or who) is your source of hope? of strength? How do they help?

To whom do you turn when you need help? Are they available?

What helps you most when you feel afraid or need special help?

How can I help you maintain your spiritual strength during this illness?

(continues)

Box 5-4. Dimensions of Spirituality with Corresponding Assessment Questions *(concluded)*

To what degree do you trust your future to God?

What brings you joy and peace in your life?

What do you believe in?

What do you do to make yourself feel alive and full of spirit?

Linkage Between Spirituality and Health

How does your spirituality affect your experience of being sick?

How has your current situation/illness influenced your faith?

How has being sick affected your sense of who you are (or how has being sick affected you spiritually)?

What has bothered you most about being sick (or in what is happening to you now)?

What do you do to heal your spirit?

Has being sick (or your current situation) made any difference in your feelings about God or your faith experience (or in what you believe)?

Is there anything especially frightening or meaningful to you now?

Do you ever wish for more faith to help you with your illness?

Has being ill ever made you feel angry, guilty, bitter, or resentful?

Sources: Inspired and adapted from Dossy, B. M. (1998). Holistic modalities & healing moments. *American Journal of Nursing, 98,* 44–47; Stoll, R. I. (1979). Guidelines for spiritual assessment. *American Journal of Nursing, 79,* 1574–1577; Dudley, J. R., Smith, C., & Millson, M. B. (1995). Unfinished business: Assessing the spiritual needs of hospice clients. *American Journal of Hospice & Palliative Care,* 12,(2), 30–37; and Alexander, W. (unpublished).

comprehensive list of questions a nurse may use for spiritual assessment. Note that these questions reflect all the major dimensions of spirituality identified in the models discussed above.

One barrier to spiritual assessment is the nurses' fear of offending a nonreligious client by using religious language. However, when one remembers the nonreligious nature of spirituality, this barrier should theoretically disappear. Client spirituality can be discussed without "God language" or reference to religion. (Box 5-4 includes numerous examples of questions without religious terms.)

To know what language will not be offensive to use during a spiritual assessment, the nurse can remember two guidelines. First, the nurse can begin the assessment with questions that are general and unrelated to religious assumptions. For example, "What is giving you the strength to cope with your illness now?" or even, "What spiritual beliefs and practices are important to you as you cope with your illness?" Second, the nurse can listen for the language of the client, and use the client's language when formulating more specific or follow-up questions. If a client responds to a question with "My faith and prayers help me," then the nurse knows "faith" and "prayer" are words that will be nonoffensive with this client. If a client states that the "Great Spirit guides," then the sensitive nurse will not respond with "Tell me how Jesus is your guide."

Use of Questionnaires

Whereas researchers often assess individuals' spirituality quantitatively with "paper-and-pencil" questionnaires, health care professionals generally assess spirituality using qualitative methods (e.g., participant observations, semistructured interviews). It is possible, however, to use questionnaires to elicit information about spirituality (O'Brien, 1999; Salisbury, Ciulla, & McSherry, 1989; Taylor, 2001; van der Poel, 1998). This approach to conducting a spiritual assessment allows for identification, codification, and possible measurement of one's spiritual beliefs and practices. Box 5-5 presents a quantitative tool for assessing spiritual status, needs, and resources. Appropriate to a variety of health care settings and contexts, this tool should not "stand alone" but should serve as a springboard for a more thorough assessment.

When using a quantitative tool, caution should be noted. The nurse must remember that such a tool should never replace human contact; instead, it should facilitate it. Also, it is possible for a client to interpret the language used in a questionnaire in a different way than would nurses. Although this is possible during a verbal interview, it is more likely to lead to miscommunication when a quantitative tool is used. When the client has completed the tool, the nurse can follow up by asking questions such as "Was there anything in the questionnaire that was confusing, or that you think could be misinterpreted?" and "Is there anything on this questionnaire that you'd especially like to discuss?'

Box 5-5. Spiritual Self-Assessment Form

Often, when people confront health challenges, they become more aware of their spirituality. For some, spiritual ways of thinking or living are especially helpful when health concerns emerge. For others, spiritual questions or doubts arise.

This form will guide you to think about spiritual issues. After completing it, you may choose to keep it or give it to your nurse, who may want to share it with other health care professionals who will be caring for you.

NAME:_____

ROOM NUMBER:_____

Place an "X" on the lines to show the answer that comes closest to describing your feelings.

Recently, my spirits have been . . .

_____

     awful. . . . . . .low. . . . . . .okay. . . . . . .good. . . . . . .great

In general, I see myself as . . .

_____

     not at all. . . . .a little. . . . .somewhat. . . . .fairly. . . . .very
     spiritual   spiritual   spiritual   spiritual spiritual

In general, I see myself as . . .

_____

     not at all. . . . .a little. . . . .somewhat. . . . .fairly. . . . .very
     religious   religious   religious religious religious

What can a nurse do that would help to nurture or boost your spirits? (check all that apply)

_____Spend quiet time with you

_____Have prayer with you

_____Help you meditate

Box 5-5. Spiritual Self-Assessment Form (continued)

_____Allow time and space for your private prayer or meditation

_____Let you know nurse(s) are praying privately for you

_____Read spiritually helpful literature to you

_____Bring art or music to you that nurtures your spirit

_____Bring you literature that you feel is spiritually helpful

_____Help you to stay connected to your spiritual community

_____Help you to observe religious practices

_____Listen to your thoughts about certain spiritual matters

_____Help you to remember how you have grown from previous diffi-cult life experiences

_____Help you to tell your life story

_____Help you to face painful questions, doubts, or suffering

_____Just be with you, not necessarily talking with you

_____Just show a genuine and personal interest in you

I would also like help in boosting my spirits from:

_____My friends and family

_____Other health care professionals

_____My own clergy or spiritual mentor

_____Other clergy or spiritual leader

_____A chaplain at this institution

What would you like your nurse to know about your prayer or meditation beliefs and practices?

_____

_____

_____

What literature, art, or music nurtures your spirit?

_____

_____

_____

(continues)

Box 5–5. Spiritual Self-Assessment Form *(continued)*

How can the nurse assist you with religious practices or fellowship?

_____

_____

_____

What spiritual matters would you like to talk about most?

_____

_____

_____

In what other ways, can the nurse help to boost your spirits?

_____

_____

_____

If there is anyone in particular you would like to meet with for spiritual fellowship, please so state. Or if there is someone you would like us to contact for you, please share what contact information you know:

_____

_____

_____

Noting Nonverbal Indicators

Although this discussion of spiritual assessment has thus far focused on how to frame a verbal question and allowing a client to verbalize a response, the wise nurse will remember that most communication occurs nonverbally. Hence, the nurse will do well to assess the nonverbal communication and the environment of the client. Chaplain John Pumphries recommends that nurses observe the ABCs of spiritual assessment (personal communication, John Pumphries, October 1986). The observer must assess the **affect, behaviors,** and **communication** of the client and determine if these elements are congruent:

- **Affect** refers to the expression of a client's emotions. Do the tone, pace, volume, pitch of voice, posture, demeanor, and other ways emotion is translated convey anger, joy, sadness, or other feelings?

- **Behaviors** are observable actions. What do activities engaged in or avoided indicate? What do gestures, body movements, and so forth convey?
- **Communication** refers to the language a client uses. What words does the client choose?

An incongruence between one's affect and words would indicate an area requiring care and further assessment. For example, the client who responds to "How are you?" with "Fine" but does so with an angry voice and eyes that look downward is demonstrating incongruency.

Another way to learn from nonverbal indicators about clients' spirituality is to assess their environment (Taylor, 2001). Are there religious objects on the bedside table? Are there religious paintings or crucifixes on the walls? "Get well" cards or books with spiritual themes? Are there indicators that the client has many friends and family providing love and a sense of community? Are the curtains closed and the bedspread pulled over the face? Does the client appear agitated or angry? And so forth. Many of the factors a nurse usually assesses will provide data for a spiritual assessment as well as the psychosocial assessment.

Family/Community Assessment

Just as an individual's spirituality influences a response to a health challenge, a family or community's response to a health or social challenge is reflective of its spirituality. Not only does spirituality influence a family or community, but it also provides coping resources. For nurses providing community-based care, a spiritual assessment can contribute invaluable information about community needs and resources. With this information the nurse can plan and provide care that ultimately impacts the spiritual health of individuals.

A home health nurse, for example, may assess a family's spirituality, or an occupational health nurse may assess the spiritual status in a corporate environment. The guidelines set forth in this chapter also apply to such assessments. Spiritual status can be assessed by asking community members to complete questionnaires or participate in focus groups where the general state of spiritual health is explored as well as perceived spiritual needs and resources. Direct observation and interviews with key informants can also be used by the nurse to survey the spiritual state of a neighborhood, corporation, religious organization, or other community. Questions to guide a community-focused assessment could include: What mission and activities provide this group of people with a sense of meaning and purpose? What religious resources exist in this community? How are they utilized by community members? What nonreligious resources spiritually nurture this community? Are there social clubs or community service organizations that foster connectedness? What do the myths and stories repeated within this family or community say about its values and beliefs? Where does this family or community turn for guidance, security, and comfort? How does this authority foster spiritual health?

Age-Appropriate Assessment Strategies

Nurses who care for clients across the life span will need to consider their stage of cognitive and spiritual development when assessing spirituality (see Chapter 1 for a discussion of spiritual development). Questions must be framed in age-appropriate language. A four-year-old, for example, will likely not understand the meaning of "spiritual resources" but may grasp, "What helps you when you're afraid?" Building trust and rapport over time with children is essential to conducting a helpful spiritual assessment (Hart & Schneider, 1997). And children are especially capable of ascertaining an adult's degree of authenticity. Children also are less likely to be offended by a question about religion. If a nurse creates a comfortable and nonjudgmental atmosphere in which a child can talk about spiritual topics, then the child will likely talk. The nurse may also need to be more creative in formulating questions if the child's vocabulary is limited. For example, instead of asking the child about "helpful religious rituals," the nurse may need to ask questions about what the child does to get ready to sleep (i.e., does he or she say a prayer at bedtime) or what the child does on weekends (i.e., attend religious services).

Young adults are in the process of identifying their own religiosity and distinguishing it from that of their parents. A nurse conducting a spiritual assessment for a young adult must be sensitive to possible cynicism and negative bias towards the religion of the previous generation. Hence, young adults will likely respond more openly to spiritual assessment questions that do not use religious language. Young adults are often searching for meaning in life and answers to deep spiritual questions. This searching may lead young adults to explore sources of comfort and meaning outside of traditional sources and institutional religion (Mabry, 1999). The nurse conducting a spiritual assessment should convey openness and remain sensitive to the searching young adult.

Older adults also have unique spiritual issues relevant to assessment
(Peterson, 1987). As people accumulate life experience, there is an
increased need to make sense of the life lived thus far, and to anticipate
death as it becomes more imminent. A method that older adults often use for
meaning making is reminiscence and storytelling. Thus, the nurse who listens carefully to shared memories can learn much about the client's spirituality. Asking specific spiritual assessment questions may not be necessary.
The nurse should also be sensitive to the fact that elders may feel some discomfort talking about spiritual issues with someone younger whom they
may perceive as incapable of understanding this dimension of life.

Communication Challenges

Although verbal conversation is integral to a typical spiritual assessment,
some clients may not be able to speak, hear, or cognitively understand a
verbal assessment. In such situations, the nurse can consult alternative
sources of information. The nurse can interview family members, observe
the client's environment and nonverbal communications. Alternative
methods for "conversing" of course can be used also. For clients who can
write, paper-and-pencil questionnaires can be very helpful (such as the
one in Box 5-5). Be prepared and unafraid of the tears which can follow
such an assessment. Clients who are unable to communicate verbally may
feel unheard. Questions that demonstrate concern for their innermost
well-being may break their floodgate for tears.

A client for whom English is a second language can also pose a challenge to the nurse trying to complete a spiritual assessment. With these
clients, a nurse can use simple drawings to determine religiosity or call a
translator. (For example, if the chart indicates the client is Roman
Catholic, the nurse can draw a picture of a church, and then have the client
point to a calendar to indicate frequency of church attendance.) When
assessing via a translator, it is important to remember that a nonprofessional translator (e.g., a family member) is likely to introduce some interpretation when translating. If this appears to be a problem, the nurse may
want to consider asking questions with yes/no responses. The nurse will
also want to carefully select the assessment questions so as to elicit maxi-
mum information with minimum questioning/translation.

Overcoming Barriers to Spiritual Assessment

Although nurses may possess the necessary knowledge for conducting a
spiritual assessment, they may still have difficulty overcoming certain bar-

riers that can interfere with spiritual assessment. These barriers include lack of time, personal discomfort with the topic of spirituality, and anxiety about how to talk with clients about the topic.

Lack of Time

Health care professionals typically believe that they do not have enough time to conduct a spiritual assessment. Maugens (1996) observed that conducting his SPIRITual history with clients took about 10 to 15 minutes, much less time than he and his colleagues expected it to take. Still, it is a considerable amount of time in today's fast-paced health care context. One simplistic response to this time barrier is to argue that nurses cannot afford not to take time to conduct a spiritual assessment, considering the fundamental and powerful nature of spirituality.

It is helpful, however, to remember that a more in-depth spiritual assessment can occur over time, in a manner which develops as the nurse gains the trust of a client. Furthermore, data for a spiritual assessment can be simultaneously collected with other assessments or during interventions (e.g., while bathing or performing bedtime care) or interaction. While a client is telling a story about her family, for example, the nurse can assess much about the client's sense of giving and receiving love and perhaps what gives meaning and purpose. While a client's spouse is describing his daily routine of caregiving, the nurse may be able to assess what provides inner strength, courage, and hope.

Nurse Discomfort

Another barrier to conducting spiritual assessment may stem from a nurse's personal discomfort with discussing spirituality with a client. Such discomfort may be expressed in statements such as, "Asking people about their spirituality is getting too personal" or "I don't want to offend anyone."

The nurse who feels discomfort assessing a client's spiritual status may lack knowledge or experience. Reading this text can counter a knowledge deficit, but the nurse may still feel uncomfortable until he or she has practiced the skill. As with inserting a nasogastric tube or any other nursing procedure, a nurse may feel some initial uneasiness until several assessments have been completed.

A nurse's spiritual experiences or unresolved spiritual needs may serve as a barrier. For example, a nurse who has an inner conflict about how to view God in relation to suffering may feel uncomfortable asking clients how illness has influenced their view of God.

Nurses inexperienced in spiritual assessment initially may feel uncomfortable raising the topic of spirituality with clients. A nurse may feel at a loss for what to ask. Memorizing a short generic question that can elicit data for a spiritual assessment (perhaps selected from Box 5-4) may help to overcome a "block."

Some nurses may believe that spirituality is an inappropriate area for nurses to address. After all, polite people do not discuss religion or politics—especially with strangers. Yet nurses customarily assess intimate areas such as elimination and sexuality. As discussed in Chapter 2, spirituality is an appropriate and necessary area for nurses to address. Hence, there is no rational explanation for this objection to spiritual assessment. It is likely that nurses who believe asking a client about spirituality is "getting too personal" are projecting their personal discomfort with the topic. If a nurse feels embarrassed performing the assessment, the client will sense that embarrassment, and may also feel embarrassed. The nurse will then perceive there is justifying evidence that conducting a spiritual assessment is too intimate a topic for a nurse–client relationship.

Some nurses may believe that "the nurse should wait for a client to raise spiritual issues." In a study of nurses' spiritual care practices and perspectives, oncology and hospice nurses responded to this statement neutrally (Taylor & Amenta, 1994; Taylor, Highfield, & Amenta, 1995). Many nurses are ambivalent about whether they should broach a spiritual topic. But considering the influence and importance of spirituality to health, nurses could be viewed as negligent if they bypassed the topic. In reality, most clients are eager to discuss their spirituality with a sensitive, caring nurse. Many are relieved when a nurse opens the topic for discussion.

Importance of Listening

Although less experienced nurses tend to focus on what to say during an assessment, the nurse must remember the importance of listening to the client's responses. Chapter 4 presents a more in-depth discussion of active listening. A few comments, however, are in order here. Remember that silence is appropriate when listening to someone's spiritual and sacred story. Listen for more than words; listen for symbols and metaphors, listen for where the client places energy, listen for feelings in addition to thoughts. The nurse will do well to listen also to his or her own inner response, because this response usually indicates the feelings of the client.

For example, the nurse listening to a client covertly expressing anger will, if aware, sense that anger internally; this awareness will then inform the nurse that the client is angry.

KEY POINTS

- Several models for spiritual assessment identify dimensions of spirituality and/or offer strategies for conducting an assessment.
- A two-tiered procedure to spiritual assessment is recommended. A focused, problem-specific assessment should follow an initial general assessment.
- Written self-report questionnaires can be used as well as verbal dialogue to assess client spiritual status, needs, and resources.
- Nonreligious and religious questions can be asked in ways that avoid discomfort.
- Spiritual assessment includes observations of client environment and nonverbal communication.
- Methods for conducting a spiritual assessment for individual clients can be applied to assessing families and communities (e.g., questionnaires, focus group interviews).
- While assessing children, young adults, or elders, the nurse needs to consider their cognitive and spiritual developmental stage and target the assessment toward the prevalent spiritual issues of their life stage.
- Clients who present with communication challenges can still be assessed using the assistance of translators, interviews with family members, and drawing and other written techniques.
- Barriers to conducting spiritual assessments include lack of time, uneasiness, and worry about what to say or ask. These barriers can be surmounted by: conducting assessments simultaneously with other nursing care, practicing, and placing the focus on listening.

LOOK WITHIN TO LEARN

1. If you find that you sometimes resist assessing a client's spirituality, what might cause you to do this? Which, if any, barriers to spiritual assessment affect your ability or willingness to assess spirituality?

2. How does it feel inside when you think about your spirituality? When you think about your own spirituality (perhaps using Box 5-4 or 5-5), what areas are easy or comfortable to think about? What areas are difficult or uncomfortable to think about? What factors might be contributing to this discomfort?

3. How does your own spirituality affect the way you relate to the spirituality of others? How might your own spirituality influence the way you approach the spiritual assessment of a client?

REFERENCES

Bold print indicates those that are most recommended.

Boutell, K. A., & Bozett, F.W. (1987). Nurses' assessment of patients' spirituality: Continuing education implications. *Journal of Continuing Education in Nursing, 21,* 172–176.

Burkhardt, M. A., & Nagai-Jacobson, M. G. (1985). Dealing with spiritual concerns of clients in the community. *Journal of Community Health Nursing, 2,* 191–198.

Carpenito, L. J. (2000). *Nursing diagnosis: Applications to clinical practice* (7th ed.). Philadelphia: Lippincott.

Dossey, B. M. (1998). Holistic modalities & healing moments. *American Journal of Nursing, 98,* 44–47.

Dudley, J. R., Smith, C., & Million, M. B. (1995). Unfinished business: Assessing the spiritual needs of hospice clients. *American Journal of Hospice & Palliative Care, 12*(2), 30–37.

Fitchett, G. (1993). *Assessing spiritual needs: A guide for caregivers.* Minneapolis: Augsberg.

Hart, D., & Schneider, D. (1997). Spiritual care for children with cancer. *Seminars in Oncology Nursing, 13,* 263–270.

Highfield, M. F., & Cason, C. (1983). Spiritual needs of patients: Are they recognized? *Cancer Nursing, 6,* 187–192.

Highfield, M. F. (1993). PLAN: A spiritual care model for every nurse. *Quality of Life, 2*(3), 80–84.

Highfield M. F. (1997). Spiritual assessment across the cancer trajectory: Methods and reflections. *Seminars Oncology Nursing, 13,* 237–241.

Hungelmann, J., Kenkel-Rossi, E., Klassen, L., & Stollenwerk, R. (1989). Development of the JAREL Spiritual Well-Being Scale. In R. M. Carroll-Johnson (Ed.), *Classification of nursing diagnoses proceedings of the eighth conference, North American Nursing Diagnosis Association* (pp. 393–398). Philadelphia: Lippincott.

Kloss, W. E. (1988). Spirituality: The will to wellness. *Harding Journal of Religion and Psychiatry, 7,* 3–8.

Koenig, H., & Pritchett, J. (1998). Religion and psychotherapy. In H. Koenig (Ed.), *Handbook of religion and mental health* (Chapter 22). San Diego, CA: Academic Press.

Mabry, J. R. (1999). The Gnostic generation: Understanding and ministering to Generation X. *Presence: The Journal of Spiritual Directors International, 5*(2), 35–47.

Maloney, H. N. (1993). Making a religious diagnosis: The use of religious assessment in pastoral care and counseling. *Pastoral Psychology, 41,* 237–246.

Maugens, T. A. (1996). The SPIRITual history. *Archives of Family Medicine, 5,* 11–16.

McSherry, W. (1996). Raising the spirits. *Nursing Times, 92*(3), 48–49.

Muncy, J. F. (1996). Muncy comprehensive spiritual assessment. *American Journal of Hospice & Palliative Care, 13,* 44–45.

O'Brien, M. E. (1999). *Spirituality in nursing: Standing on holy ground.* Boston: Jones and Bartlett.

Peterson, E. A. (1987). How to meet your clients' spiritual needs. *Journal of Psychosocial Nursing, 25,* 34–39.

Pruyser, P. W. (1976). *The minister as diagnostician.* Philadelphia: Westminster Press.

Reed, P. G. (1987). Spirituality and well-being in terminally ill hospitalized adults. *Research in Nursing & Health, 10,* 335–344.

Salisbury, S. R., Ciulla, M. R., & McSherry, E. (1989). Clinical management reporting and objective diagnostic instruments for spiritual assessment in spinal cord injury patients. *Journal of Health Care Chaplaincy, 2,* 5–64.

Stoll, R. I. (1979). Guidelines for spiritual assessment. *American Journal of Nursing, 79,* 1574–1577.

Taylor, E. J. (2001). Spiritual assessment. In B. Ferrell & N. Coyle (Eds.), *Textbook of palliative nursing care* (pp. 379–406). New York: Oxford University Press.

Taylor, E. J., & Amenta, M. O. (1994). Midwifery to the soul while the body dies: Spiritual care among hospice nurses. *American Journal of Hospice & Palliative Care, 11*(6), 28–35.

Taylor, E. J., Amenta, M. O., & Highfield, M. F. (1995). Spiritual care practices of oncology nurses. *Oncology Nursing Forum, 22,* 31–39.

VandeCreek, L., Ayres, S., & Bassham, M. (1995). Using INSPIRIT to conduct spiritual assessments. *Journal of Pastoral Care, 49*(4), 83–89.

van der Poel, C. J. (1998). *Sharing the journey: Spiritual assessment and pastoral response to persons with incurable illnesses.* Collegeville, MN: Liturgical Press.

Yeadon, B. E. (1986). Spiritual assessment for a community-based hospice. *Caring, 5*(10), 72–75.

6

Nursing Care for Spiritual Needs

The quintessence of nursing is caring. Nursing care strives to be holistic, providing clients with support and nurture for their physiologic, emotional, and spiritual needs. The nursing process, an organized approach to caring, guides nurses to assess, identify client strengths and needs, determine appropriate outcomes and develop a plan to achieve them, and implement interventions and evaluate their effectiveness. Because effective nursing care addresses client spirituality, which is an integral aspect of health and well-being, the nursing process is a helpful way to approach spiritual caregiving.

After completing an assessment and before planning interventions for any health challenge, the nurse must formulate a diagnosis that identifies the needs of the client and, if possible, determine their etiology. Not only does a diagnosis offer a label that helps health care professionals to communicate easily, but a diagnosis and recognition of its etiology help to determine appropriate nursing interventions. If, for example, a woman who complains of nausea is incorrectly diagnosed in the emergency room, she may be treated for a bowel obstruction when her condition warrants treatment for pregnancy.

Accurate diagnosis is similarly vital with a spiritual health challenge. If a client's spiritual need is not diagnosed, professional interventions will not ensue. If a client's spiritual need is diagnosed with insufficient specificity or without recognition of its etiology, the interventions will likely be inappropriate, ineffective, and possibly harmful. And if the diagnosis and resulting plan of care is not documented, the spiritual care will not be well coordinated or complete. The purpose of this chapter, therefore, is to present key elements of nursing care to promote spiritual health: diagnosing, planning, implementing, and evaluating as well as strategies for documenting spiritual care.

DIAGNOSING SPIRITUAL NEEDS

Nurses, as well as physicians, mental health professionals, and chaplains/pastoral counselors, are aware of the helpfulness of formulating correct and precise diagnoses for clients with spiritual needs (Carpenito, 2000; Kelly, 1995; Maloney, 1993; Turner, Lukoff, Barnhouse, & Lu, 1994). Although as summarized in Box 6-1, various diagnostic labels for spiritual needs have been recommended, most nurses subscribe to the approach developed by the North American Nursing Diagnosis Association (NANDA), which recognized spiritual needs as early as 1978.

NANDA (1999) recommends three diagnoses specific to spiritual need: spiritual distress, potential for enhanced spiritual well-being, and risk for spiritual distress.

Spiritual Distress

Spiritual distress is "a disruption in the life principle that pervades a person's entire being and that integrates and transcends one's biological and psychological nature" (NANDA, 1999, p. 67). Spiritual distress (i.e., distress of the human spirit) refers to any disruption—or dis-ease—in one's spirit. This diagnostic label could apply to clients who report that their

Box 6-1. Diagnostic Labels Indicating Spiritual Need		
Author	**Label**	**Comments**
NANDA (Carpenito, 2000)	(a) Spiritual distress (b) Potential for enhanced spiritual well-being	Spiritual distress can be specified as related to: (a) (Specify [e.g., immobility, depression, hospitalization]), as evidenced by inability to practice spiritual rituals (b) Conflict between religious or spiritual beliefs and prescribed health regimen (c) Crisis of illness, suffering, or death
American Psychiatric Association (Turner et al., 1995)	Religious problem (e.g., change in denominational affiliation, intensification of adherence to beliefs or practices, loss or questioning of faith, guilt, cult membership) Spiritual problem (e.g., lack of integration related to a mystical experience, near-death, or terminal illness; spiritual emergency)	This diagnostic category was added to the 4th edition of the *Diagnostic and Statistical Manual of Mental Disorders* (DSM-IV) published in 1994; it is listed under "Other Conditions That May Be a Focus of Clinical Attention"

(continues)

| Box 6-1. Diagnostic Labels Indicating Spiritual Need *(continued)* |

Author	Label	Comments
O'Brien (2000)	(a) Spiritual pain (b) Spiritual alienation (c) Spiritual anxiety (d) Spiritual guilt (e) Spiritual anger (f) Spiritual loss (g) Spiritual despair	Introduces these diagnoses as being related to "alterations in spiritual integrity"
Hay (1989)	(a) Spiritual suffering (b) Inner resource deficiency (c) Belief system problem (d) Religious need	Each defined as: (a) Interpersonal and/or intrapsychic anguish of unspecified origin (b) Diminished spiritual capacity (e.g., low level of that which empowers, animates; low aspirations) (c) Lack of conscious awareness of personal meaning system (d) Specifically expressed religious request

"spirits are down" or they feel "broken-hearted." Such indicators may reflect a range of spiritual concerns, including client feelings of abandonment by God or by others, or doubts about religious or spiritual beliefs. Box 6-2 summarizes defining characteristics for this diagnosis. Examples of NANDA diagnoses that address spiritual distress include:

Box 6-2. Defining Characteristics for Spiritual Distress

- Expresses concern with meaning of life/death and/or belief systems
- Questions moral/ethical implications of therapeutic regimen
- Description of nightmares/sleep disturbances
- Verbalizes inner conflict about beliefs
- Verbalizes concern about relationship with deity
- Unable to participate in usual religious practices
- Seeks spiritual assistance
- Questions meaning of suffering
- Questions meaning of own existence
- Displacement of anger toward religious representatives
- Anger toward God
- Alteration in behavior/mood evidenced by anger, crying, withdrawal, preoccupation, anxiety, hostility, apathy, etc.
- Gallows humor

Source: NANDA. (1999). *Nursing diagnoses: Definitions and classification 1999–2000.*
Philadelphia: Author.

- Spiritual distress related to searching for meaning of illness as manifested by voicing of "why me?" questions.
- Spiritual distress related to quest for purpose in life and self-worth as manifested by the statement, "Now that I'm confined to a wheelchair, what good am I?"
- Spiritual distress related to inability to participate in religious practices (i.e., unable to attend mosque or perform ritual Islamic prayers and ablutions) as evidenced by the remark, "I feel like I am disobedient to Allah's commands when I can't kneel to prayer like usual."

Potential for Enhanced Spiritual Well-Being

Identified as a diagnosis by NANDA in 1994, "potential for enhanced spiritual well-being" recognizes that "spiritual well-being is the process of an individual's developing/unfolding of mystery through harmonious interconnectedness that springs from inner strengths" (NANDA, 1999, p. 68). This diagnosis acknowledges client desire to attain a higher level of spiritual wellness and may be appropriate when clients manifest inner strength, peace, joy, a sense of purpose, respect for mystery and challenges in life, or harmonious connections with others, the world, and their Ultimate Other. Examples of this diagnosis include:

- Potential for enhanced spiritual well-being related to facing imminent death as manifested by the statement: "It's strange, but having cancer has made me a better person. Now that I know I'm going to die young, I want to work to leave a legacy."
- Potential for enhanced spiritual well-being related to unknown etiology as manifested by comment, "I want to feel closer to my heart, more aware of my spiritual core."
- Potential for enhanced spiritual well-being related to surviving a serious illness as evidenced by the statement, "I should be dead now, but I'm not. There must be a purpose for my life and I am going to find out what it is."

Risk for Spiritual Distress   1998

"Risk for spiritual distress" was defined in 1998 by NANDA as being "at risk for an altered sense of harmonious connectedness with all of life and the universe in which dimensions that transcend and empower the self may be disrupted" (NANDA, 1999, p. 68). This diagnosis may be appropriate for a client who presently shows no indication of this disruption of spirit yet may if a nurse fails to intervene. A client coping with a disease or illness that will eventually cause physical pain is at risk for spiritual distress because such pain often arouses spiritual questions like "why me?" and "where is God when I suffer?" A victim of violence may also be at risk for spiritual distress because responses to victimization often include doubts about self-worth or the goodness of other people, issues of forgiveness, and so forth. Box 6-3 summarizes risk factors. Examples of NANDA diagnoses that address risk for spiritual distress include:

- Risk for spiritual distress related to immobility and inability to attend synagogue weekly as evidenced by the appearance of sadness and

---

Box 6-3. Risk Factors for Spiritual Distress

- Blocks to self-love
- Energy-consuming anxiety
- Inability to forgive
- Loss of loved one
- Low self-esteem
- Maturational losses
- Mental illness
- Natural disasters
- Physical illness
- Physical or psychological stress
- Poor relationships
- Situation losses
- Substance abuse

Source: NANDA. (1999). *Nursing diagnoses: Definitions and classification 1999–2000.*
Philadelphia: Author.

---

statements like "I know I'm going to miss the closeness I feel with God if I can't worship like I normally do on Shabbat."

- Risk for spiritual distress related to inability to forgive self as manifested by cynical comments and statements like "I knew better, so why did I smoke? I was such a weakling! Guess I have to learn to forgive myself for smoking."

Beyond those specific to spiritual health, other NANDA diagnoses also identify needs linked to spiritual well-being. Diagnoses that describe client conditions which may carry underlying distress of the human spirit, summarized in Box 6-4, alert the nurse to the presence of spiritual needs. A client diagnosed with body image disturbance related to facial burns, for example, may be angry at God for allowing the injury to occur and may wonder if others can feel comfortable around her. Thus, spiritual care may be an important element in planning interventions to address diagnoses linked to spiritual well-being.

Box 6-4. Nursing Diagnoses Often Accompanied by Spiritual Distress

- Altered role performance
- Anticipatory or dysfunctional grieving
- Body image disturbance
- Chronic sorrow
- Death anxiety
- Decisional conflict
- Defensive coping
- Fear
- Hopelessness
- Impaired social interaction
- Ineffective (or potential for enhanced) coping (specify individual, family, or community)
- Noncompliance
- Powerlessness
- Risk for loneliness
- Risk for self-mutilation
- Self-esteem disturbance
- Social isolation

Research Implications

NANDA nursing diagnoses related to spirituality were formulated based on existent nursing knowledge during the 1980s and 1990s. Subsequently, a few nurse researchers have studied the validity of the diagnosis "spiritual distress." Research has assisted in the determination of defining characteristics which indicate spiritual distress (Hensley, 1994; McHolm, 1991; Weatherall & Creason, 1987). Although studies validate the diagnosis of spiritual distress, they suggest that defining attributes may need further refinement. Pehler (1997) attempted to validate the diagnosis for use with children. In this study, an expert panel of chaplains suggested that NANDA's defining characteristics of spiritual distress were more likely to accurately indicate spiritual distress among older teens than among children. Pehler observed that some indicators of spiritual distress among children are absent from the NANDA list (e.g., issues of fairness, fear of the future or the unknown, frustration).

Heliker (1992) argued that the diagnosis of spiritual distress lacked the discriminatory power, generality, and flexibility necessary for a useful diagnostic label. To enhance diagnostic reasoning, Heliker suggested that nurses must be able to view spirituality as broader than religiousness and to appreciate various cultural and philosophical perspectives on spiritual belief. Engebretson (1996) identified three Western spiritual assumptions that may bias nursing views of spirituality and even contribute to misdiagnosis: monotheism (i.e., assumption that there is one God); dualism (i.e., that body and spirit are separate); and thinking that transcendence refers only to connecting with spiritual entities beyond the self.

Because they are relatively recent additions to the NANDA list, risk for spiritual distress and potential or enhanced spiritual well-being have not as yet been systematically studied and need to be empirically validated. Many studies undertaken to validate spiritual distress have serious methodological limitations (e.g., failure to include a non-Western perspective; small sample sizes; use of methods that involve only nurses rather than including other experts like clients or chaplains to evaluate the defining characteristics.) Future research can address these limitations and enhance findings by studying large, diverse samples (e.g., people of all ages and cultural backgrounds).

Some in nursing have resisted taxonomizing and diagnosing client health challenges, especially those that arise in connection with spirituality. Mayer (1992) questioned whether spiritual needs should be subjected to diagnosis:

> It is pertinent to keep questioning the assumption that spirituality can be classified and controlled, quantified and written up in nursing notes, and processed in such a way that questions about ultimate values and intimate areas of relationship can be asked, answered, and recorded in the same way as questions about fluid balances, bowel function, and body chemistry. And if it is deemed to be possible, then further questions need to be asked about whether it should be. (p. 33)

Mayer's sensitivity to the intangible nature of spirituality suggests that it may be difficult to communicate client spiritual concerns using traditional documentation methods.

Diagnosing actual or potential spiritual needs helps to ensure that they are acknowledged and addressed. Using standardized, specific terminology (such as NANDA's) may increase the chance that clinicians will plan and implement spiritual care in a systematic and effective manner. Failing to make such a diagnosis, likewise, may increase the chance that nurses will miss an opportunity to comfort and aid healing.

PLANNING SPIRITUAL CARE

After formulating a diagnosis that identifies a client's spiritual health needs, the nurse creates a plan for providing spiritual care. Planning activities include determining desired outcomes and selecting appropriate nursing interventions. Box 6-5 presents a sample care plan.

Box 6-5. Nursing Care Plan: Mr. Goddard's Spiritual Distress

Mr. Goddard, a 54-year-old business executive with renal cell cancer who identifies himself as an agnostic, is admitted for chemotherapy. He appears to be anxious and asks, "What do you think happens to people when they die?"

Spiritual Assessment Focus: End-of-life concerns and beliefs about afterlife, coping strategies for addressing death anxiety

Nursing Diagnosis: Spiritual distress related to uncertainty about beliefs regarding death and afterlife

Expected Outcomes & Outcome Evaluation	Nursing Interventions
Decreased dissatisfaction or uncertainty with beliefs regarding death and afterlife (e.g., will verbalize increased satisfaction or feeling of peace about beliefs)	• Encourage verbalization regarding spiritual beliefs about death by asking open-ended questions to promote inner awareness (e.g., "Tell me about how your beliefs about death have changed during your life.") • Provide strength for introspection about death and afterlife by practicing presence.

Box 6-5. Nursing Care Plan: Mr. Goddard's Spiritual Distress *(continued)*	

Expected Outcomes & Outcome Evaluation	Nursing Interventions
Decreased sense of death anxiety (e.g., will identify at least one comforting coping strategy)	• If requested, make a referral to a chaplain. (Chaplain may make a referral to a clergyperson with beliefs similar to those described by the client.) • Encourage client to discuss feelings or dreams (e.g., "What have you learned from your fears about dying?" "Have you been having any troubling dreams?") • Explain intense feelings are appropriate and informative. • Help client to determine coping strategies that have been helpful during previous life transitions; determine strategies that will be most effective now. • Facilitate coping strategies selected (e.g., teach or provide instructional material on meditation, provide writing materials for art or journal writing). • If requested, make referral to psychotherapist, art or music therapist.

Because spiritual health reflects and contributes to physiologic and emotional health, the diagnosis of spiritual distress should generally receive high priority in the plan of care. Often, however, this diagnosis is not accorded the priority it deserves. A medical orientation that emphasizes physiologic processes and the discomfort of some care providers with spirituality and spiritual caregiving may explain the lower priority.

Standardized goals for nursing plans are being developed in nursing (Kozier, Erb, Berman, & Burke, 2000). The Nursing Outcomes Classification system identifies the goal for the diagnosis of spiritual distress as "spiritual well-being." This broad objective allows much flexibility, within which the nurse can incorporate more specific and measurable desired outcomes. Nurse researchers have also identified and organized nursing interventions. The Iowa Nursing Interventions Classification list includes interventions for "spiritual support." Whether or not the nurse elects to use a nursing taxonomy to plan care to address spiritual needs, interventions must reflect the uniqueness of the client, specifics of the diagnosis, and etiology of the problem.

Brennan (1997) identified several challenges that arise when identifying outcomes and interventions. Improvements in spiritual health may not be achieved within predictable time frames or in a predictable manner. It would obviously be unrealistic, for example, to enter in the client's plan of care plan that he or she "will stop asking 'why me?' within 3 days." Brennan suggested that improving spiritual well-being is a process. How well it moves forward may depend on the nurse's ability to practice presencing. Within the time the nurse provides care, this process may or may not support the client to achieve a satisfactory level of spiritual well-being. Mayer (1992) also points out that it is impossible and inappropriate for nurses to devise care plans that attempt to control and fix client spiritual needs. Interventions chosen to support spiritual well-being will often, therefore, emphasize facilitating the process of greater spiritual awareness rather than a concrete, measurable goal.

Box 6-6 provides another example of a care plan developed to address a client's spiritual needs. Comparing the plan in Box 6-5 with that in Box 6-6 will reveal how interventions for clients with spiritual distress can greatly differ, depending on the etiology of the distress.

NURSING INTERVENTIONS FOR SPIRITUAL CAREGIVING

Although developing a plan of care requires the nurse to identify interventions, the term *interventions* is often inappropriate when applied to spiritual care (Mayer, 1992). Interventions suggest doing, rather than being, and imply that one who intervenes is superior, charged with fixing someone who is inferior. Spiritual care, however, typically involves being (rather than doing) and striving for symmetry in the nurse–client relationship. In the absence of a more suitable term, *interventions* will be used to refer to nursing approaches to the provision of spiritual care.

When caring for a client with spiritual needs, the nurse can utilize various interventions identified in nursing literature (Kozier et al., 2000; Taylor

Box 6-6. Nursing Care Plan: Ms. Khan's Spiritual Distress

Ms. Khan, an unmarried 22-year-old college student, has miscarried a five-month pregnancy. As she is prepared for a dilation and curettage (D&C), she angrily remarks, "I know God is punishing me." Although her parents are Moslem, she has not participated in any religion for five years.

Spiritual Assessment Focus: Perceptions about the nature of God and how God relates to persons, beliefs about punishment and how they apply to her, feelings of loss and grief (e.g., of fetus, of innocence, of happiness)

Nursing Diagnosis: Spiritual distress related to guilt about premarital sex and grief about miscarriage

Expected Outcomes & Outcome Evaluation	Nursing Interventions
Elimination of sense of guilt (e.g., will verbalize sense of forgiveness) Movement toward increased positive regard for God (e.g., will verbalize decreased feelings of anger toward self and God) Decreased feelings of anger and sadness (e.g., appears more restful, peaceful)	• Encourage open expression of guilt by presencing and active listening • Assist client to create (and perhaps implement) a meaningful ritual that signifies cleansing and forgiveness • Encourage client to explore forgiveness by God and self (e.g., in journal, in dialogue with spiritual mentor) • Encourage exploration of beliefs about God's character and ways of relating to humans (e.g., in journal, in dialogue with spiritual mentor).* • Facilitate expression of feelings of loss by practicing presence • Explore usefulness of coping strategies (e.g., journal writing, meditation, crying, talking with friends or God or counselor) • Assist client to consider positive outcome(s) from this painful experience, to identify some meaning

*Helpful questions include: Who/what is God like to you? What has influenced this way of viewing God? How is God loving/hateful? How do you think God relates to people? Like a parent, teacher, psychologist, or governor? How is your God like your parents? What informs you about what is wrong behavior? How do you think God relates to people who do wrong things? How does your God want to relate to you? How do you want to relate to God?

Box 6-7 Interventions for Spiritual Care

- Active listening
- Bibliotherapy (reading spiritually uplifting materials, including sacred writings)
- Caring touch
- Dream analysis
- Expressive art (e.g., music, sculpture, painting, knitting, dance)
- Facilitating religious practices
- Facilitating social support
- Humor
- Imagery
- Journal writing or scrapbook making
- Meditation
- Nature
- Praying with or for clients or assisting clients to pray
- Presencing
- Referral to spiritual care expert for counseling or instruction
- Story listening and storytelling, reminiscence, or life review

& Mickley, 1997). The complexity and varieties of spiritual needs of diverse clients certainly requires numerous approaches to spiritual care. A partial list of interventions that can boost the spirit are presented in Box 6-7. The nurse uses sensitivity to select or develop interventions that will achieve expected outcomes and promote spiritual health. Interventions should be based on scientific knowledge and professional standards of care. They should also reflect philosophical or theological perspectives of the client, without compromising those of the nurse. Because spiritual care typically involves "being with," effective interventions encourage client involvement.

EVALUATING EFFECTIVENESS OF SPIRITUAL CARE

When evaluating spiritual care, criteria to determine effectiveness center on how well desired outcomes have been achieved. It is important to remember that it is the client's—not the nurse's—desired outcome that should constitute the standard. Although some outcomes of spiritual care will be measurable (e.g., attendance at religious services once every week or initiation of an expressive art project), many will be less concrete. Increased spiritual well-being may sometimes be observed overtly. A client, for example, may appear less anxious or at peace, may have become more open and comfortable speaking about a spiritual need, or may openly verbalize awareness of increased spiritual health.

In the process of moving toward an increased sense of spiritual health, many clients may experience spiritual "growing pains" such as the discomfort of being emotionally challenged while contemplating doubt, the mental fatigue that results when trying to make sense of a loss or change, or the challenge of learning spiritual discipline (e.g., learning to meditate for more than two minutes). A client who experiences such spiritual discomfort is traveling a path toward spiritual healing and health and is likely making significant progress toward attaining a desired outcome.

DOCUMENTING SPIRITUAL CARE

The adage about documentation, "if it was not charted, it was not done," applies also to spiritual care. Documenting spiritual care serves several purposes. It allows health care professionals to communicate with one another about client spiritual needs that have been identified, interventions that have been helpful, and client responses to spiritual care. Documentation supports auditing and quality assurance and provides researchers and analysts with information that can ultimately lead to improvements in health care.

Various documentation systems are currently in use. Health care organizations, especially acute care settings, are increasingly adopting systems that require minimal effort and time (e.g., charting by exception, flowsheets). Although any format or system can be used to document spiritual caregiving, this section will focus on strategies that require minimal nursing time.

The Joint Commission on Accreditation of Healthcare Organizations (JCAHO) requires health care organizations to document the assessment of spirituality. Most hospital admission forms ask fewer than three brief questions about spirituality. These forms typically request information about client religious affiliation, desire for a chaplain visit, and client spiritual practices about which the health care team should be sensitive. Often, admission forms ask if there is a spiritual concern that the client perceives. These questions usually are formatted with yes/no and short fill-in-the-blank response options that allow the nurse to rapidly document an initial spiritual assessment.

Hospices and hospitals affiliated with a religious organization often provide a more thorough system for documenting information about client spirituality. Checklists with potential spiritual strengths and concerns allow a nurse or spiritual care expert to quickly and precisely document information. Computerized charting with screens that trigger a more in-depth spiritual assessment form or written charting with an optional spiritual assessment form can be used to document more detail when a spiritual diagnosis is evident.

A personalized spiritual care plan is ideal, but sometimes nurses need to rely on a standardized plan of care. Standardized care plans save nursing time, providing a list of expected outcomes for the nurse to check as appropriate. Most address spiritual distress, but many omit the diagnoses of potential for enhanced spiritual well-being or risk for spiritual distress. Standardized care plans that provide space to add "other" information can compensate for the uniform format.

Spiritual care interventions and client responses to them can also be documented efficiently. Some institutions have developed checklists of spiritual care interventions that nurses can use to record care they have provided. Sometimes interventions are categorized as spiritual interventions or religious sacramental services. Some forms include a checklist of client responses. Again, documentation forms that allow a nurse to enter "comments" encourage flexibility and support individualized care.

Box 6-8 presents an example of a standardized spiritual care plan, designed to address diverse needs across a broad range of health care settings. It would be appropriate to streamline this plan by identifying those spiritual needs most frequently encountered in a particular setting. The spiritual needs of hospice patients, for example, will generally differ from those of clients admitted to intensive care units. This plan of care, therefore, can be adapted to meet setting-specific client needs. While this care plan offers three sections (i.e., for diagnoses, expected outcomes, and interventions), additional institution-specific formatting for charting dates, nurse initials, and other information can be incorporated.

Box 6-8. Standardized Care Plan for Spiritual Needs

Directions: Check each problem, outcome, or intervention you determine to be appropriate for the client. Add further information as needed.

Nursing Diagnoses

- ❏ Spiritual distress . . .
- ❏ Risk for spiritual distress . . .
- ❏ Potential for enhanced spiritual well-being . . .

Related to . . .

- ❏ Expressed concern with meaning of suffering or death
- ❏ Expressed concern about personal purpose or mission
- ❏ Need to give/return love or express care to others
- ❏ Need to feel love from others, participate in community
- ❏ Need for love, self-worth, dignity (from self/God)
- ❏ Challenged world assumptions or spiritual beliefs
- ❏ Questions about ethics of therapeutic regimen
- ❏ Frustration or anger at self, others, or God
- ❏ Need for hope, peace, or joy
- ❏ Boredom and need to express creativity
- ❏ Doubt about, or sense of insecurity or distance from deity
- ❏ Difficulty engaging in religious rituals (e.g., prayer) due to spiritual/emotional reasons
- ❏ Inability to participate in religious practices due to physical disability
- ❏ Disconnection/conflict with faith community
- ❏ Disconnection/conflict with loved ones
- ❏ Need for forgiveness or reconciliation (with God or others)
- ❏ Anxiety about, or fear of:
- ❏ Questions about making right choices (e.g, ethical dilemma)
- ❏ Other:

(continues)

Box 6-8. Standardized Care Plan for Spiritual Needs *(continued)*

Please explain your diagnosis or provide information about how this diagnosis is manifested:

Expected Outcomes & Outcome Criteria

❑ Expresses increased satisfaction with spiritual coping strategies

❑ Expresses movement toward satisfactory answers or meanings

❑ Expresses increased awareness of spiritual need/s or spiritual self-awareness

❑ Expresses awareness of being loved or of ways to give love

❑ Renews participation in religious practices or community

❑ Identification of personal spiritual care plan and methods for implementing it

❑ Verbalizes less anxiety or fear or appears peaceful

❑ Reports experiencing increased sense of harmony/closeness with self, others, nature, or deity

❑ Identifies healthful ways for expressing the soul, joy, or creativity

❑ Perceives positive visit from spiritual care expert

❑ Other:

Explain further as necessary:

Nursing Interventions

❑ Practice presencing

❑ Active listening

❑ Introduce helpful questions; identify areas for focus:

❑ Facilitate religious practices; please specify:

❑ Pray with or for clients, or assist to pray

❑ Refer to spiritual care expert; please specify:

❑ Story listening, reminiscence, or life review

❑ Teach or facilitate meditation or imagery

❑ Provide restful nature experiences

Box 6-8. Standardized Care Plan for Spiritual Needs *(concluded)*

❏ Facilitate soul expression through art; please specify client preference:

❏ Introduce humor appropriately

❏ Provide guidance for dream analysis

❏ Bibliotherapy; specify reading material(s) and method:

❏ Encourage/facilitate expression of thoughts and feelings via journal writing or scrapbook making

❏ Provide caring touch during procedures and at other times

❏ Facilitate social support

❏ Other:

Please provide additional details about appropriate interventions tailored to client needs:

KEY POINTS

- Various diagnostic labels for spiritual needs have been created by experts, the most widely used generated by NANDA. NANDA diagnoses include spiritual distress (or distress of the human spirit), risk for spiritual distress, and potential for enhanced spiritual well-being.

- Spiritual distress refers to disruption in the principle that pervades a client's life, or dis-ease in a client's spirit.

- Potential for enhanced spiritual well-being is a nursing diagnosis that recognizes a client's process of becoming more spiritually healthy as well as the desire for a higher level of spiritual wellness.

- Risk for spiritual distress is a nursing diagnosis appropriate for a client who presently shows no indication of this disruption of spirit, yet may if a nurse fails to intervene.

- Nursing diagnoses that do not specify spirituality (e.g., body image disturbance, chronic sorrow) may still reflect spiritual needs. Incorporating these needs within the plan of care promotes client well-being.

- Although studies validate the diagnosis of spiritual distress, they suggest that defining attributes may need further refinement.
- Although developing a care plan personalized for each client is preferable, standardized spiritual care plans provide an efficient method for establishing baseline data as well as recording individualized information.
- Effective spiritual care involves selecting interventions that are specific to the needs and uniqueness of the client.
- Documentation allows members of the health care team to communicate with one another about the process and outcomes of spiritual care and supports the continuing study of spiritual caregiving.

LOOK WITHIN TO LEARN

1. How will your diagnosis of a spiritual need influence the care you provide?

2. How might what you document in an initial assessment influence the degree to which spiritual care is provided during a client's admission?

3. Your client has a spiritual need to express joy at the birth of a long hoped for child (or upon receiving welcome news that has ruled out a serious health problem). Using the Standardized Care Plan (Box 6-8), which nursing diagnosis would you select? Which outcomes and interventions might be appropriate? How might you individualize care for your client?

4. If you indicate in your verbal nursing report a diagnosis of spiritual distress and the observation that your client appreciates prayer but fail to document these things, how might client care be affected?

REFERENCES

Bold print indicates those that are most recommended.

Brennan, M. R. (1997). Spiritual distress/Potential for enhanced spiritual well-being. In G. K. McFarland & E. A. McFarlane (Eds.), *Nursing diagnosis & intervention: Planning for patient care* (3rd ed.). (pp. 852–862). St. Louis, MO: Mosby.

Carpenito, L. J. (2000). *Nursing diagnoses: Application to clinical practice* (8th ed.). Philadelphia: Lippincott.

Engebretson, J. (1996). Considerations in diagnosing in the spiritual domain. *Nursing Diagnosis, 7*(3), 100–107.

Hay, M. W. (1989). Principles of building assessment tools. *The American Journal of Hospice Care, 6*, 25–31.

Heliker, D. (1992). Reevaluation of a nursing diagnosis: Spiritual distress. *Nursing Forum, 27*(4), 15–20.

Hensley, L. D. (1994). Spiritual distress: A validation study. In R. M. Carroll-Johnson & M. Paquette (Eds.), *Classification of nursing diagnoses: Proceedings of the tenth conference* (pp. 200–202). Philadelphia: Lippincott.

Highfield, M. F., & Cason, C. (1983). Spiritual needs of patients: Are they recognized? *Cancer Nursing, 6,* **187–192.**

Kelly, E. W., Jr. (1995). *Spirituality and religion in counseling and psychotherapy: Diversity in theory and practice.* Alexandria, VA: American Counseling Association.

Kozier, B., Erb, G., Berman, A. J., & Burke, K. (2000). *Fundamentals of nursing: Concepts, process, and practice* (6th ed.). Upper Saddle River, NJ: Prentice Hall Health.

Maloney, H. N. (1993). Making a religious diagnosis: The use of religious assessment in pastoral care and counseling. *Pastoral Psychology, 41,* 237–246.

Mayer, J. (1992). Wholly responsible for a part, or partly responsible for a whole? The concept of spiritual care in nursing. *Second Opinion, 17*(3), 26–55.

McHolm, F. A. (1991). A nursing diagnosis validation study: Defining characteristics of spiritual distress. In R. M. Carroll-Johnson (Ed.), *Classification of nursing diagnoses: Proceedings of the ninth conference* (pp. 112–119). Philadelphia: Lippincott.

North American Nursing Diagnosis Association. (1999). Nursing diagnoses: Definitions and classification 1999–2000. Philadelphia: Author.

Pehler, S. (1997). Children's spiritual response: Validation of the nursing diagnosis spiritual distress. *Nursing Diagnosis, 8*(2)**, 55–66.**

Taylor, E. J., & Mickley, J. R. (1997). Introduction. *Seminars in Oncology Nursing, 13,* 223–224.

Turner, R. P., Lukoff, D., Barnhouse, R. T., & Lu, F. G. (1994). Religious or spiritual problem: A culturally sensitive diagnostic category in the DSM-IV. *The Journal of Nervous and Mental Disease, 183,* **435–444.**

Weatherall, J., & Creason, N. S. (1987). Validation of the nursing diagnosis, spiritual distress. In A. M. McLane (Ed.), *Classification of nursing diagnoses: Proceedings of the seventh conference* (pp. 112–119). St. Louis: Mosby.

7

Spiritual Support for Clients Searching for Meaning

Many persons for whom nurses provide care experience deep spiritual pain related to questions about why bad things happen. The following excerpt illustrates many points about the process of searching for meaning:

At first I was just afraid and very tearful. I never said "why me?" or "why has this happened to me?" I used to wonder why bad things kept happening to me. But now I just feel that there is no rationale for most things— bad things just happen in general, and that's part of the life experience. You find you have a heck of a lot of strength that you never knew you had. It's amazing how strong it's [fighting cancer] has made me feel. So I think

*a lot of it is meeting the challenge. Buddhists say that all life is sorrow.
And I think that's right; I think that there are good things and bad things
that just happen. And I could have sat there and cried for the rest of my
life or just gotten on with it, and getting on with it is what I chose to do.
I'm just not going to die over sadness from the disease. I'm going to live
my life and have a life, and if the disease gets me, it gets me.*

—*43-year-old woman living with stage IV breast cancer*

Negative, unexpected life events often shatter clients' beliefs and precipitate
the asking, as this woman does, of a "why?" question. This process, wherein
people "try on" an array of answers to find those that "fit," frequently leads
to recognition of spiritual growth. This chapter explores dimensions of
searching for meaning that clients experience and presents nursing
responses to support clients who experience this form of spiritual distress.

DEFINING SUFFERING

Suffering is a human response to various life experiences. Illness, with its
accompanying physical, emotional, relational, and spiritual components,
often precipitates suffering. Suffering, which differs from physiologic
pain, may hurt much more than pain. A frequently cited definition recognizes that suffering occurs when clients perceive a threat to or the destruction or disintegration of their personhood (Cassel, 1982). Cassel (1991)
also proposed that suffering can occur only if someone is self-aware, conscious of time, and able to think about the future.

Reich (1989) described suffering as:

*An anguish which we experience on one level as a threat to our compo-
sure, our integrity, and the fulfillment of our intentions but at a deeper
level as a frustration to the concrete meaning that we have found in our
personal existence. It is the anguish over the injury or threat of injury to
the self—and thus to the meaning of the self—that is at the core of suffering. (p. 85)*

Suffering does not necessarily occur in the presence of uncontrolled
severe pain but when that pain is viewed as meaningless, unfair, or a
deterrent to accomplishing life goals. Suffering is also present when a
client experiences fatigue if it prevents socializing, knitting, or other
activities that contribute to maintaining a sense of identity, self-worth, or
community.

SEARCHING FOR MEANING THROUGH QUESTIONING

When people, particularly those influenced by Western worldviews (Mohrmann, Healey, & Childress, 2000), experience or witness suffering, unsettling questions will often arise. Why do bad things happen, especially to good people? Does evil exist, or do bad things just happen? Often, such questions will incorporate a theological dimension: If God is loving, then why does suffering occur? If God is all powerful, why isn't evil contained? Such questions illustrate the problem of theodicy, or the need to defend God's ways. Theologians who address the problem of theodicy are attempting to answer the question "How can God's ways be justified?" (Harper, 1990).

When confronted with personal suffering, clients who do not believe in a God or an Absolute may also struggle with existential or philosophical questions. Clients coping with illness or disability may question whether there is any order or fairness in the universe. Or they may ask questions not only about the purpose of life but also about the purpose of their lives (Thompson & Janigian, 1988; Taylor, 1995). Those with terminal illness often wonder what occurs after death.

Process of Searching for Meaning

Social psychologists observe that individuals naturally respond to negative, unexpected life events with questions about meaning (e.g., Janoff-Bulman, 1992; Tedeschi & Calhoun, 1995). People generally adopt a set of assumptions about themselves and their world, assuming the world to be benevolent and meaningful and people to have worth. Traumatic events such as a debilitating accident, loss of a child, or diagnosis of a serious illness can shatter such assumptions. When people's assumptions about the world are damaged, their struggle to cope with the trauma often leads them to reconstruct their world view to adopt a wiser, more encompassing outlook. This struggle involves balancing the act of thinking about the painful subject with that of avoiding painful thoughts—a process of approach/avoidance (Janoff-Bulman, 1992).

Research findings suggest that most but not all persons with serious health challenges will acknowledge some sort of search for meaning. Taylor (1993a) observed that the act of searching for meaning when illness struck did not always result in finding a satisfactory meaning. The search for meaning is conceived by many researchers as a process. Ferrell and colleagues (1993) proposed that the process of attributing meaning to cancer pain followed an order: first, immediate causes are identified (e.g., "the pain means I have cancer"); second, the immediate effects are recognized (e.g., "the pain means I can't do the things I used to do"); and last, ultimate causes are proposed by the sufferer (e.g., "the pain is God's will").

Taylor (2000) described the process that women experienced in order to attribute significance to the diagnosis of breast cancer. Participants initially "encountered darkness" by acknowledging dark, difficult, and psychospiritually painful questions that they were drawn to ask of themselves. Next, they "converted darkness" by accepting that some of their questions were unanswerable and by choosing to live beyond the questions. Doing this allowed these women to "encounter light" or perceive the positive benefits introduced to them by their illness. Finally, this experience allowed them to "reflect light" or to demonstrate in visible ways their inner transformation. Taylor's metaphorical labels for these four phases were inspired by the comments of one informant: "I think the search for meaning is finding light in the darkness or finding a greater perspective that can bring peace" (p. 783).

Types of Questions

Questions that arise when people seek to understand an unfortunate experience can take different forms. Thompson (1991) suggested three categories of attributions:

- Causal attributions (e.g., "What caused this to happen?" "Why do bad things like this happen?")
- Selective incidence attributions (e.g., "Why me?" "Why did this happen to me instead of to someone else?")
- Responsibility attributions (e.g., "Is God, chance, or the environment to blame for this happening to me?" "Did I do anything to cause this to happen to me?" "What is it about me that made this happen?")

Taylor (1995) suggested an additional type of attribution sometimes raised by seriously ill clients that relates to significance. Instead of focusing on the cause of a misfortune, the client may be drawn to consider its beneficial impact on the future. This ability to transform a health-related tragedy into something positive has been observed among many persons who suffer (Tedeschi & Calhoun, 1995; Park, 1998; Barasch, 1993) and led Moch (1989) to posit that this kind of transformation is what allows for "health within illness."

Many clients will convert the "why me?" question to "why not me?" (e.g., "This could have happened to anybody, why not me?"). Taylor (1995) observed that those who ask this "why not me?" question appear to find some relief from the spiritual distress of asking "why me?" perhaps because their search for meaning is supported by their assumption that tragedy happens randomly.

Barriers to Client Disclosure

Although theory and research suggest that clients experiencing traumatic life events are likely to pose "why?" questions in their search for meaning, they may not always voice these concerns to nurses at the bedside. Several factors may discourage client disclosure:

- The client may lack sufficient courage to ask "why me?" or "how do I transform this tragedy?" It may be difficult for clients to voice questions for which they do not know—or may fear—the answer.
- Some clients harbor questions but perceive that pondering them is unhelpful or a waste of time.
- The nurse may unwittingly convey the message that expression of such painful questions is personally discomforting. Clients often "test the waters" to see if the nurse is someone worthy of trusting with their inner thoughts. A nurse who responds with statements like "Oh, don't be so serious" or "Don't worry, everything is going to be okay" or attempts to impose personal beliefs would likely fail this test.
- The client may have been conditioned to avoid or deny questions of meaning and thus may refrain from verbalizing them. Some religiously oriented clients believe it is sinful to entertain "why?" questions, because the act of questioning is perceived as an inappropriate challenge of God's will.
- Clients may raise questions indirectly, initially denying that they are struggling to resolve questions. When they are encouraged to talk about their inner experience, these issues may emerge. As the cancer survivor in the introduction illustrated, "I never said 'why me?'. . . [but wondered] why bad things keep happening to me."
- For some clients, the search for meaning is not conducted consciously. The nurse may recognize the search for meaning embedded in a client's conversation. A description of life events may be an attempt to establish life purpose and legacy. A reflective statement such as "if it happened, then it must have happened for a reason" may indicate searching. In a less direct manner, these are attempts to construe meaningfulness.

APPROACHES TO MAKING MEANING

Science has generated valid answers to many questions about the causes of wellness and disease—answers that tend to satisfy clients. Answers to questions prompted by suffering, however, are ultimately unprovable, and it is human to wrestle with such questions. Various approaches to making meaning allow clients to cope with their suffering. While some approaches tend to involve thinking, others involve doing. Whether cognitive, behavioral, or theological—or whether hypothetical or scientifically supported—interpretations that make suffering meaningful provide comfort.

Cognitive and Behavioral Approaches

The ways in which clients answer their own "why?" questions in order to cope and gain perspective have been recorded by social psychologists, nurses, and other health care researchers (e.g., Taylor, 2000; Janoff-Bulman, 1992; Thompson, 1991; Foley, 1988). In one of the first studies on this topic, Janoff-Bulman and Wortman (1977) observed six categories of responses to the "why me?" question among clients who experienced recent spinal cord injuries: predetermination ("It was fate"); probability ("The statistics support this happening to me"); chance ("It was a completely random event"); "God had a reason"; deservedness ("I am being punished"); and positive benefit ("This has made me a better person"). Similar categories have been observed subsequently among other samples of persons experiencing illness. Foley (1988) interviewed clients visiting a chronic pain clinic to ascertain how they interpreted their suffering and categorized their responses as summarized in Box 7-1.

In order to investigate how victims of a home fire approached the process of finding meaning, Thompson (1985) reviewed empirical and journalistic literature and identified five ways people reevaluate an experience as positive:

1. Identifying side benefits (e.g., "It was good that this happened, because it made our family draw closer together.")
2. Making social comparisons (e.g., "My neighbor was so much worse off.")
3. Imagining worse situations (e.g., "It could have been worse—I could have died.")
4. Forgetting the negative (e.g., "I blanked it out.")
5. Redefining ("Now I'm content if I my pain is only mild.")

Box 7-1. Interpretations of Suffering (Foley, 1988)

Interpretation	Example
Punishment	"I am sick because I sinned and disobeyed God."
Testing	"My illness is a test of my faith. Although God doesn't give us more than we can bear, I resent being tested."
Bad luck	"It was just my luck to get sick." *Fatalistic belief*
Submission to the laws of nature	"You just have to grin and bear it." "I just need to be patient and let nature take her course."
Resignation to the will of God	"It's God's will. I can't figure out why, but God let it happen for some reason—maybe."
Acceptance of the human condition *humanism (to be flawed)*	"I choose to actively engage in life, even though I know my illness will kill me. I have a purpose for living until the end comes. While I hope for a miracle, I realize that I may experience a lot of suffering."
Personal growth *educational*	"God is trying to teach me something through this suffering."
Defensiveness and denial	"I think it is better to ignore suffering and just try to forget it."
Minimization *putting things into perspective*	"At least my situation isn't as bad as my neighbor's."
Divine perspective	"This disability isn't God's will; but God does give it meaning. As I reflect, I see it as a blessing in disguise."
Redemption *Martin Luther King*	"I can actually rejoice in my suffering, because I am understanding and sharing in Christ's suffering, life and death." *participate*

Source: Adapted from Foley, D. P. (1988). Eleven interpretations of personal suffering. *Journal of Religion and Health, 27,* 321–328.

Others have suggested that, in addition to these cognitive strategies, self-blame may assist in reconstructing shattered assumptions (Janoff-Bulman, 1992). For example, a client who states, "Because it was my fault, I can prevent it from happening again" is able to cling to some sense of control in a seemingly uncontrollable world.

Research documenting the positive meaning that clients attribute to their health challenges is increasing. No longer is the focus limited to the negative psychosocial sequelae of illness. Rather, there is evidence suggesting that illness and other traumatic life events can produce a positive transformation for clients (Park, 1998; Tedeschi & Calhoun, 1995) Taylor's (2000) qualitative study reported outcomes for this illness-induced transformation among breast cancer survivors. These outcomes are illustrated in Box 7-2 and suggest positive meanings that clients can construe for illness.

Box 7-2. Research Profile: Transformation of Tragedy Among Women Surviving Breast Cancer

- **Purpose:** To describe the process and outcomes of attributing positive meanings to the experience of breast cancer.

- **Methods:** Descriptive, qualitative methods including in-depth semi-structured interviews with 24 women surviving breast cancer.

- **Main Findings:** Several categories of positive meaning (or significance) that women ascribed to their illness were identified. These included:

  - Reevaluation and Reprioritization of Personal Values (e.g., "I've realized how unimportant 'toys' are, having money and things like that; and how important my friends are, and my family. It's put it all in very clear perspective now.")

  - [Re]consideration of Life Direction and Mission (e.g., "I think I needed to make an adjustment in my life at this point, and maybe the cancer brought the focus to do it. . . . I needed to examine where I was and how I got there. . . . I think that it [cancer] has made me decide what my purpose was and has helped me to define the things that I feel I need to do in my life.")

  - Urgency and Immediacy About Life, Causing One to Live with Intentionality, in the Present (e.g., "It has really given me a better

---

(continues)

Box 7-2. Research Profile: Transformation of Tragedy Among Women Surviving Breast Cancer (continued)

knowledge of what it means to live one day at a time, what it means to appreciate what you have right now." "I feel now that when I do things, I do them for a reason.")

- Profound Appreciation of Life and Nature (e.g., "I see things in a much more positive light. I get up in the morning and I'm glad there's a new day [crying]. And, I'm more thankful for my family and definitely more aware of the beauty around me . . . there is a greater sense of joy in everything. Whether it's being with family, experiences at work, or just walking around and seeing the flowers and the birds and that sort of thing.")

- Intensified Spiritual Awareness, Often Accompanied by Inner Peace (e.g., "I'm closer to my heart." "It has changed me. Spiritually, I'm more in tune and more aware of God and what He has planned for me. It truly is a spiritual experience.")

- Increased Self-Knowledge and Self-Respect (e.g., "I'm a better person than I thought I was for myself. I'm more satisfied with me than caring about what somebody else is feeling about me. . . . It's making me have to take care of myself, be patient, and not rush around in a hurry.")

- Healthy Perspective About Self in Relation to Others and the World (e.g., "I've done this housecleaning with people who are leeches on my emotions, and on the energy that I have to spend. . . . Before, I'd say yes when I didn't mean to say yes, then I'd be angry that I had to do it; now I just say no." "I realize now that my number one priority is taking good care of myself. I also realized that I had numerous friends and so many people who care deeply about me, something I failed to recognize before.")

- Nursing Implications: A client can ascribe positive meanings to cancer without necessarily understanding its cause. By helping clients to recognize the necessity and importance of "encountering the darkness," the nurse can support the client in the process of making meaning.

Source: Tayler, E. J. (2000). Transformation of tragedy among women surviving breast cancer. *Oncology Nursing Fourm, 27,* 781–788.

Yalom (1980) identified a variety of "secular activities" that assist people who suffer to derive a sense of meaning. He categorizes them as follows:

- Altruism (i.e., serving others, leaving the world a better place)
- Dedication to a cause (whether it be a political, family, state, or religious cause)
- Creativity (i.e., creating something new—be it artistic or scientific—that is beautiful, unique, or harmonious)
- Hedonism (i.e., engaging in activities that allow one to live life to the fullest)
- Self-actualization (developing the self's fullest potential)
- Self-transcendence (placing one's focus away from the self).

Frankl (1986) proposed three ways in which people can find meaning. First, there is what one gives to the world. Second, meaning can be found through what one takes from the world. Third, Frankl submitted that the ultimate way of finding meaning is through the attitude one chooses to take in the face of suffering. According to Frankl (1984), a person can find meaning through the following:

- Tasks (actualized by doing; e.g., helping others, work)
- Creative or aesthetic experiential moments that bring meaningfulness (e.g., watching a sunset from a mountaintop, listening to moving music, or feeling an embrace)
- Attitudinal values (i.e., when faced with unalterable suffering, a person formulates an attitude that gives suffering meaning).

Religious Approaches

Those who believe in God may find that their belief is challenged when they experience suffering. Mohrmann (in Mohrmann et al., 2000) suggests three ways in which persons resolve their struggle to make sense of suffering in relation to God:

You can change what you believe about God, or even whether you believe, in order to devise a way to make sense of the inescapable reality of the suffering and to recreate some kind of order. Or, you can change what you believe about the suffering, even about its reality, so that you make it fit somehow with what you still believe about God. Or, of course, you can do a little of each. (p. 60)

A client who is diagnosed with a severely debilitating disease may, for example, decide that God does not exist or that God is uninvolved or unconcerned about his welfare. More likely, however, this client will wonder what he did to deserve the disease, or he may opt to believe that the disease is a blessing in some way. Mohrmann's observation is similar to those of psychologists who have suggested that persons maintain cognitive control when responding to negative events by either redefining their view of the world, the event, or their view of themselves.

It is the life work of many theologians and philosophers to theorize about the meaning of loss, illness, suffering, and other unfortunate events. Misfortune is usually explained by theologians in ways that do not change the assumptions that God is powerful and loving; rather, they reinterpret suffering in a way that fits these assumptions about God (Mohrmann et al., 2000). Vicchio (1989) suggested categories that capture how religion explains suffering. The following are adapted from those he proposed and reflect explanations frequently encountered:

- **Punishment.** A cause-and-effect relationship exists between sin and its consequences. If one does not obey God's laws of health, for example, sickness can result. Thus, bad things happen because one has sinned, been bad, and deserves this punishment.
- **Consequence.** The "free will defense" reasons that God created humans to have free wills—to respond to and obey God's love and laws. Because it would be unloving and incongruent with God's nature to force obedience, and because of the human proclivity to disobey, suffering occurs as a consequence.
- **Benefit.** One explanation proposes that misfortune and suffering benefit people by bringing out their moral good qualities. To gain these prized qualities, God allowed or created a world with misfortune. Another aspect of this teleological explanation for suffering posits that in the future there will be harmony and perspective that provides meaning for current temporal sufferings (e.g., "when we get to Heaven we'll see how all things worked together for good").

For many clients, religious beliefs provide immense comfort, positive meaning, and a healing way to relate to suffering. Suffering can be a door for spiritual growth. Religion can assist this passage toward inner transformation. This is evidenced by the research that demonstrates a positive correlation between religiousness and health, and the helpful role religiosity plays in coping (see Chapter 10).

NURSING IMPLICATIONS

Eliminating or reducing suffering is a fundamental goal of nursing care. Beyond this goal, a profound outcome for someone who suffers may be the opportunity to experience spiritual growth or transformation. Such an experience cannot be engineered by the nurse. It is rather a gift that the nurse may be privileged to help convey. The nurse who is able to facilitate a healthy spiritual response to suffering is typically someone who is adept in the process of spiritual caregiving. Effective care of the spirit requires the ability to develop and integrate many of the spiritual care strategies discussed in this text, such as empathic listening, compassionate touch, presencing, supportive prayer, promoting religious practices that comfort, and so forth. Additional suggestions for practice pertinent to searching for meaning follow.

Being Present

Arguably the most important ways the nurse can support a suffering client are to remain present and to receive the story of suffering. Being present, however, requires that nurses recognize and attend to their own spiritual anxieties and suffering. The ability to be present and receptive to another's suffering derives from a state of inner calm. When sufferers recount their story, often in fragmented pieces that may seem no longer to fit (e.g., their assumptions about life, their losses, their beliefs about the Divine, their doubts and questions, their hopes, their devastation), nurses through their compassionate presence can offer support by "holding" these fragments (Bouchard, 1999).

Encouraging Resiliency

Another strategy for supporting those who suffer is to teach that the spirit is resilient. How can nurses encourage resiliency? They might consider several approaches to helping clients to learn that the spirit is resilient. Nurses can inform clients that others in similar circumstances have construed positive meaning and benefits from experiences of loss, illness, or disability. It may be helpful to remind clients that even though painful, the process of searching for meaning is normal. Nurses can share insights but need to do so without pushiness. For example, the nurse might say:

I sense that you may be feeling upset about how you are suffering. If it is helpful to you, I would like you to know that others in similar circum-

stances have told me that they were eventually able to discover positive aspects of the experience. With time, you may share this outcome.

The nurse can assist a client to recall earlier challenging life events that led to positive transformation. Recalling how they may have benefited from having survived a previous illness or crisis may inspire clients to gain the courage to believe that they will in some way "be the better" for the current misfortune.

The nurse may want to suggest an inspiring role model. Clients may draw strength from someone who in similar circumstances surmounted suffering. A cancer survivor, for example, may develop inner resilience from the experiences of a friend or relative or from reading the autobiography of Gilda Radner (the celebrity who lived authentically and humorously with cancer).

Encouraging Client Disclosure

Asking thoughtful questions and listening attentively to responses may help the client to gain awareness. Examples include:

- What are some of the good things that have come out of your loss/illness/disability experience?
- What sorts of lessons about life have you learned from this experience?
- What have you learned about yourself through this current crisis?
- How has this experience affected your sense of purpose or mission in life?

Theologian Patricia Wismer (1995) recommended that spiritual care providers encourage clients to embrace ambiguity:

Instead of pretending to answer the unanswerable, I propose that we follow the advice of German poet Rainer Maria Rilke and simply "live the question." We need, Rilke says, to: ". . . be patient towards all that is unsolved . . . and try to love the questions themselves. . . . Live the questions now. Perhaps you will then gradually, without noticing it, live along some distant day into the answer." (p. 149)

Consider, for example, how to respond to a client who states, "I've been a good person all my life. Why would this happen to me?" The sensitive nurse could say something like, "I understand that questions like this can be incredibly painful, but I'd like to encourage you to stay with the question as much as you are able. From what I understand, questions like this can lead to greater understanding." The nurse might follow with one or more of the above questions as a catalyst for continuing the process of finding positive meaning.

Wismer (1995) recommended the following question as helpful: Who suffers with me/you? Recognizing that others, a deity, or the client's community or "web of life" share the suffering can be comforting. Encouraging clients who suffer to perceive that they are not alone is generally helpful. It is possible, however, to initially compound a client's suffering with such a question if the client responds with "Nobody suffers with me." The nurse's ministry of presence can be a powerful antidote for client feelings of being alone in suffering.

Responding Appropriately

Sensitive spiritual care avoids addressing unanswerable questions with superficial answers. Inappropriate responses include:

- "God doesn't give you more than you can bear." (The client may feel that the degree of suffering *is* more than he or she can bear.)
- "This is a test of your faith; be glad that God loves you so!" (Although the client may be comforted to be reminded of a loving deity, comments such as this may convey an unsettling perspective of a sinister deity.)
- "It must be God's will." (Statements like this often represent an attempt to avoid complex subjects.)
- "There is a reason this happened. Probably because. . . ." (Avoid imposing personal beliefs on the spiritually vulnerable client.)
- "There are no answers, so asking questions won't help." (Avoid trying to dodge the client's need to express the pain.)

Strategies to Facilitate Making Meaning

Yalom (1980) identified specific strategies for making meaning, illustrated in Box 7-3.

The ability to facilitate the attainment of satisfactory explanations for why suffering occurs still does not erase suffering (Hauerwas, 1990). Theology and philosophy offer abstract, paradigmatic ideas about the problem of suffering. Theorizing with clients about their suffering does

Box 7-3. Strategies for Making Meaning	
Strategy	**Example**
Altruism	Volunteering (e.g., reading stories to children)
	Participating in research (to help others who currently or in the future will confront a similar loss/illness/disease)
	Providing kindness (e.g., writing letters to prison inmates, giving flowers to fellow patients)
	Leaving a legacy (e.g., telling your story, creating something by which your family, friends, or the world can remember you)
Dedication to a cause	Political (e.g., campaigning for health care or insurance reform by making phone calls or writing letters to Congress or newspapers)
	Social (e.g., assisting with literacy or environmental projects)
	Religious (e.g., involvement in church projects or committees)
Creativity	Artistic (e.g., writing prose or music about the illness experience, making a scrapbook, making toys for babies with AIDS)
	Scientific (e.g., inventing a chair that helps patients with dyspnea, researching the literature regarding a symptom you observe in yourself and other patients)
Hedonism	Appreciating relationships with friends and family
	Enjoying the beauty of nature and art (e.g., listening to a Brahms symphony, going to the beach, savoring favorite foods)
Self-actualization	Individual psychotherapy
	Introspection and journaling
Self-transcendence	Praying (especially for others)
	Meditating

Source: Taylor, E. J. (1993). The search for meaning among persons with cancer. *Quality of Life—A Nursing Challenge, 2*(3), 65–70. Courtesy Meniscus Health Care Communications.

not eliminate suffering. Hauerwas contended that suffering is lessened to some degree by allowing the sufferer to "name the silences." Naming silent pains (e.g., doubts or hurts that are hard to talk about) helps to reduce their oppressiveness.

Psychological Adaptation to Suffering

Research about how clients attempt to attribute a cause or meaning to an illness indicates that persons who are actively searching, or are stuck searching, have poorer psychological adaptation to that illness (Taylor, 1993a; Lowery, Jacobsen, & DuCette, 1993). A client who says "I know there's got to be a reason for this happening to me, but I just can't figure it out!" may be experiencing difficulty in adjusting. Thus, introducing questions of causality and meaning to clients who have not directly or indirectly alluded to searching may be detrimental to their adaptation.

Although clients who are actively searching for meaning may have greater psychological maladaptation, those who have progressed through the process of reconstructing meaning appear to be grateful for what they perceive to be a life transformation (Taylor, 2000; Tedeschi & Calhoun, 1995). Nurses should therefore avoid discouraging clients who are drawn to engage in this process. When clients verbalize questions about their suffering, the effective nurse demonstrates an appreciation for the value inherent in the asking. Instead of avoiding clients or dismissing their questions, the nurse should respond with openness. Confronting the "darkness" of suffering appears to be requisite to experiencing the "light" that suffering may also bring (Taylor, 2000).

Although much of the literature suggests that suffering can inspire positive meaning and even transform a person spiritually, Smolkin (1989) argued that a time can arise when painful experiences no longer function "redemptively," as indicated by the following criteria: (1) when the client can no longer plan a course of action, (2) when the client can no longer learn from the painful experience, and (3) when the client can no longer take measures to change anything. In situations like these, effective spiritual care focuses on presencing, building or sustaining a sense of community for the client, and prayer (Oates, 1974).

The client who suffers, regardless of the circumstances that cause or contribute to suffering, provides an opportunity for the nurse to demonstrate caring competence. Box 7-4, a plan of care for a client experiencing suffering, summarizes nursing interventions to assist the client to alleviate and transform suffering.

Box 7-4. Nursing Care Plan: Mrs. Lee and Johnny

Johnny Lee, age 21, is admitted to the hospital for the fourth time for sickle cell pain crisis. At his bedside, his mother, Mrs. Lee, finds it difficult to console John. While discussing his pain management protocol with the nurse, she asks, "Why does my son have to suffer so much? It's not fair!"

Nursing Diagnosis: Spiritual distress related to search for meaning amidst physical suffering

Expected Outcomes & Outcome Evaluation	Nursing Interventions
Participation in meaningful activity and verbal recognition of construed benefits	Encourage the client and his mother to describe their search for meaning, either verbally, through expressive art, or journal writing. If appropriate, suggest open-ended questions to prompt inner exploration (e.g., If you could ask the Creator questions, what would they be? [If journal writing, suggest that clients write their questions with their dominant hand, and whatever response they sense with their nondominant hand.])
	Especially during times when physical pain is uncontrolled, provide presencing (or coordinate a schedule of volunteers, chaplains, family, and friends to provide presence).
	At times when pain is more controlled, encourage the client to explore what positive outcomes or benefits have come from his health challenge (e.g., ask "What good things have resulted from having an illness?").
	Assess the client's life mission or purpose. Explore with the client how this mission can continue or be redirected. Encourage/facilitate activities that remind the client of "the bigger picture" (e.g., letter writing, visiting or helping another client, praying for nurses or others with pain)

Box 7-4. Nursing Care Plan: Mrs. Lee and Johnny *(continued)*

Nursing Diagnosis: Potential for enhanced spiritual well-being related to the opportunity to transform tragedy

Expected Outcomes & Outcome Evaluation	Nursing Interventions
Verbalized indication of movement toward transformation	Use presencing and active listening to show support as the client names "silent pains" and encounters the sometimes dark, disturbing questions of meaning.
	Conduct a life challenges review (elicit stories from the client's life about previous life challenges and how they were surmounted)
	Encourage/facilitate discussion of religious responses to suffering with an appropriate spiritual care expert.
	Introduce the client to another for whom sickle cell or other painful condition prompted spiritual transformation (e.g., a biography about this "hero").

KEY POINTS

- Pain, suffering, and traumatic life events may shatter assumptions that clients hold about their world and lead them to search for meaning.

- The search for meaning can occur at various levels and may manifest by the need to pose different types of questions (e.g., attributions of causality, selective incidence, blame and responsibility, and questions about significance).

- Questions raised by clients who suffer often relate to theodicy, a theological term that refers to the difficulty of reconciling the existence of a good and powerful God with the reality of suffering.

- Research has documented various client responses to ways in which clients respond to their own questions about meaning.

- A variety of approaches to assist clients to construct meaning are available to nurses, including:

○ Teaching that the spirit is resilient (e.g., reviewing positive personal growth resulting from previous negative life experiences).

○ Asking helpful questions to assist the client to increase awareness of positive meaning previously derived.

○ Respecting the client's need to question and helping them to "live the questions."

○ Refraining from providing superficial answers (especially to ultimately unanswerable questions).

○ Suggesting the question "Who suffers with you?" and exploring the comfort of others, God, or the client's community or "web of life."

○ Introducing clients to various cognitive and behavioral strategies that create a sense of meaning.

○ Refraining from exploring the topic unless the client directly or indirectly raises the issue.

LOOK WITHIN TO LEARN

1. How do you explain the reality of suffering or why bad things happen to people? Which beliefs from Box 7-1 resonate with you?

2. Have any negative life experiences shaped your beliefs about the world or yourself? In what ways have they changed you for the better?

3. How secure are you in your spiritual beliefs? Would a negative life event shatter your assumptions and faith? (What if you became a quadriplegic after a car accident? What if one of your parents died suddenly? What if you were diagnosed with leukemia?)

4. How would you relate to a client who held different conclusions about suffering or "God's will?" How would you take care not to impose on a client your understanding of why bad things happen?

5. Review the statement by the woman with breast cancer that opened this chapter. In what ways did this client search for meaning? What answer(s) did she find that she felt to be satisfactory? As her nurse, how might you have assisted her with this process of creating meaning?

REFERENCES

Bold print indicates those that are most recommended.

Barasch, M. I. (1993). *The healing path: A soul approach to illness*. New York: Putnam.

Bouchard, L. D. (1999). Holding fragments. In M. E. Mohrmann & M. J. Hanson (Eds.), *Pain seeking understanding: Suffering, medicine, and faith*. Cleveland, OH: Pilgrim Press.

Cassel, E. J. (1982). The nature of suffering and the goals of medicine. *New England Journal of Medicine, 306*, 639–645.

Cassel, E. J. (1991). Recognizing suffering. *Hastings Center Report, 21*(3), 24–31.

Ferrell, B., Taylor, E. J., Sattler, G., Fowler, M., & Chency, B. L. (1993). Searching for the meaning of pain: Cancer patients; caregivers; and nurses' perspectice. *Cancer Practice, 1*(3), 185–194.

Foley, D. P. (1988). Eleven interpretations of personal suffering. *Journal of Religion and Health, 27*, 321–328.

Frankl, V. (1984). *Man's search for meaning*. New York: Washington Square Press.

Frankl, V. (1986). *The doctor and the soul*. New York: Vintage Books.

Harper, A. W. J. (1990). *The theodicy of suffering*. San Francisco: Mellen Research University Press.

Hauerwas, S. (1990). *Naming the silences: God, medicine, and the problem of suffering*. Grand Rapids, MI: Eerdmans.

Janoff-Bulman, R. (1992). *Shattered assumptions: Towards a new psychology of trauma*. New York: Free Press.

Janoff-Bulman, R., & Wortman, C. (1977). Attributions of blame and coping in the "real world": Severe accident victims react to their lot. *Journal of Personality and Social Psychology, 35*, 351–363.

Lowery, B. J., Jacobsen, B. S., & DuCette, J. (1993). Causal attributions, coping strategies, and adjustment to breast cancer. *Journal of Psychosocial Oncology, 10*(4), 37–53.

Moch, S. D. (1989). Health within illness: Conceptual evolution and practice possibilities. *Advances in Nursing Science, 11*(4), 23–31.

Mohrmann, M. E., Healey, D. E., & Childress, M. D. (2000). Suffering's witness: The problem of evil in medical practice. *Second Opinion, 3*, 55–70.

Oates, W. E. (1974). *Pastoral counseling*. Philadelphia: Westminster Press.

Park, C. L. (1998). Stress-related growth and thriving through coping: The roles of personality and cognitive processes. *Journal of Social Issues, 54*, 267–277.

Reich, W. T. (1989). Speaking of suffering: A moral account of compassion. *Soundings, 72*(1), 83–108.

Smolkin, M. T. (1989). *Understanding pain: Interpretation and philosophy*. Malabar, FL: R. E. Krieger.

Taylor, E. J. (1993a). Factors associated with meaning in life among people with recurrent cancer. *Oncology Nursing Forum, 20*, 1399–1407.

Taylor, E. J. (1993b). The search for meaning among persons with cancer. *Quality of Life—A Nursing Challenge, 2*(3), 65–70.

Taylor, E. J. (1995). Whys and wherefores: Adult perspectives of the meaning of cancer. *Seminars in Oncology Nursing, 11*(1), 32–40.

Taylor, E. J. (2000). Transformation of tragedy among women surviving breast cancer. *Oncology Nursing Forum, 27*, 781–788.

Tedeschi, R. G., & Calhoun, L. G. (1995). *Trauma and transformation: Growth in the aftermath of suffering*. Thousand Oaks, CA: Sage.

Thompson, S. (1985). Finding meaning in a stressful event. *Basic and Applied Social Psychology, 6*, 279–295.

Thompson, S., & Janigian, A. S. (1988). Life schemes: A framework for understanding the search for meaning. *Journal of Social and Clinical Psychology, 7*, 260–280.

Thompson, S. C. (1991). The search for meaning following a stroke. *Basic and Applied Social Psychology, 12*(1), 81–96.

Vicchio, S. J. (1989). *The voice from the whirlwind: The problem of evil and the modern world.* Westminster, MD: Christian Classics.

Wismer, P. (1995). For women in pain: A feminist theology of suffering. In A. O. Graff (Ed.), *In the embrace of God: Feminist approaches to theological anthropology.* Maryknoll, NY: Orbis Books.

Yalom, I. D. (1980). *Existential psychotherapy*. New York: Basic Books.

8

The Role of the Nurse in Collaborating with Spiritual Care Professionals

Whereas some nurses consider themselves to be experts in a particular area of health care delivery, others have expertise as coordinators of health care. When it comes to providing spiritual care, most nurses are generalists rather than specialists. Thus, the purpose of this chapter is to explore how nurses as generalists in spiritual caregiving can effectively collaborate with professionals who are specialists in spiritual care. Such collaboration provides clients with the benefits of a multidisciplinary team—knowledge, support, and resources from professionals whose services complement the care of nurses.

NURSES AS SPIRITUAL CARE GENERALISTS

Naturally, there are various levels of clinical competence in spiritual care-giving among nurses. Because of their own personal attentiveness to spiritual matters, some nurses are inherently able to provide spiritual care. Others have acquired spiritual care skills through various informal and formal instructional programs or academic education. Some nurses, for example, acquire knowledge from chaplaincy training or graduate programs in pastoral counseling or ministry. Most nurses, however, have not participated in such programs.

It is not unusual for nurses to consider their religious instruction or attendance at religious services as training for spiritual caregiving (Highfield, Taylor, & Amenta, 2000). Although a religious background can provide a nurse with sensitivity toward spiritual needs and caring interventions, it is also possible that nurses may inappropriately introduce their own religiosity when attempting to provide spiritual care. As presented in Chapter 3, spiritual care that imposes the nurse's religious views and overlooks the client's spiritual needs is unethical and potentially harmful.

In fact, the majority of nurses perceive themselves to be fairly religious (Taylor, Highfield, & Amenta, 1999; Scott, Grzybowski, & Webb, 1994; McSherry, 1998). Professional nursing organizations and federal data sets do not collect information about the religiosity of nurses. A few studies with a large sample of U.S. nurses, however, have included religiosity as one of the demographic variables (Scott, Grzybowski, & Webb, 1994; Taylor & Amenta, 1994; Taylor, Highfield, & Amenta, 1994). These studies typically found that about 90 percent of all respondents identify themselves as Christian, and about 10 percent identify another religion (e.g., Judaism, Buddhism) or see themselves as nonreligious. When comparing these findings with those from polling of a large U.S. sample (Gallup, 1996), there is evidence that the religiosity of nurses may differ somewhat from that of the general population. The likelihood of claiming membership in a formal religion is the same, and 69 percent of nurses did so. However, nurses may be more likely to attend religious services weekly (40 to 50 percent of nurses versus 31 percent of general population), and are more likely to be Roman Catholic (about 35 to 40 percent of nurses versus 25 percent of general population). These findings, albeit based on limited samples, demonstrate that religion does influence the personhood—and consequently, practice—of many nurses.

SPECIALISTS IN SPIRITUAL CARE

Professionals who have received training and formal education in spiritual care, pastoral counseling, theology and psychology, chaplaincy, and so forth are typically considered to be the experts in spiritual care. Shamans, medicine men, curanderos (or curanderas), and other folk healers, however, may also be considered spiritual care experts by many clients from non-Western cultures. Just as nurses refer clients with significant family or economic problems to a social worker, clients with disabilities that affect activities of daily living to an occupational therapist, and clients with swallowing problems to a speech therapist, so also should a nurse refer a client with significant spiritual needs to a spiritual care specialist.

Consultations with spiritual care experts are generally free of charge. Chaplain services, like nursing services, are included in general hospital or home health charges. Clergy are paid by ecclesiastical sources, as are many parish nurses and spiritual directors. There are a variety of specialists who may be experts in spiritual care. By understanding the different backgrounds and roles of these specialists, the nurse can choose the most appropriate specialist for the referral.

Chaplains

Professional chaplains can provide invaluable support to address the spiritual needs of clients and also of nurses. The field of chaplaincy reflects a merger of theology and psychology. Those trained in chaplaincy have a good understanding of how to help persons with health-related transitions or challenges who use spiritual beliefs and practices. An estimated 9,000 U.S. chaplains belong to at least one of four professional chaplaincy organizations (personal communication, Larry VandeCreek, Director, Pastoral Research, HealthCare Chaplaincy Association, May 30, 2000). Although it is unknown how many health care institutions employ a chaplain, the Joint Commission on Accreditation of Healthcare Organizations (JCAHO) requires that institutions make formal arrangements for chaplaincy services. Whereas some institutions hire professional chaplains, others use the services of volunteer chaplains and clergy.

Professional chaplains can receive certification from at least three different professional organizations. To become certified, a chaplain must have completed a full year of Basic Clinical Pastoral Education (CPE; i.e., 1,600 hours, which are divided among 4 units) or an equivalent experience, and possibly an additional year of advanced CPE residency. CPE provides the chaplain intern with didactic instruction, individual and group supervision, and practicum. An important goal for chaplain interns during CPE is that of understanding "the use of self as a spiritual tool in ministry" (Association of Professional Chaplains, 2000). For certification, chaplains must also possess a graduate degree in theology or ministry, be recognized as a clergyperson by their religious denomination, and be endorsed by a faith group for ministry as a chaplain (Association of Professional Chaplains).

Many chaplains are highly skilled professionals. Not all who serve as chaplains in health care settings, however, have received formal training. Many chaplains are actually clergy or laypersons who volunteer their services to the health care institution. In addition to a staff chaplain, most hospital chaplaincy departments recruit volunteer chaplains from the religions represented by the client population. These unpaid chaplains typically have not received any CPE.

Nurses consult chaplains to support a variety of client spiritual needs. Scott and colleagues (1994) found that the most common reasons for a nurse–chaplain consultation were:

- Family support in times of death and emergencies
- Arrangement of bedside religious rites
- Anxious or fearful client
- Family support for difficult decision making
- Cessation of life support
- Do not resuscitate decisions
- Spiritual needs assessment

The preceding functions exemplify the four broad roles of chaplains identified by chaplains VandeCreek, Carl, and Parker (1998). These include conducting spiritual assessments of clients, responding to clients' religious concerns and helping them with religious coping strategies (e.g., understanding biblical stories, leading worship experiences), supporting professional staff, and functioning as a liaison with religious communities by being a representative of religion.

Hospital chaplains typically see nurses and other hospital staff as their parishioners. They can be a resource for the nurse personally as well as professionally. For example, chaplains have facilitated support groups to assist nurses with coping with the many stressors of work. Chaplains also often counsel nurses individually about work-related issues, marriage and family problems, or other personal problems. Chaplains perform marriage ceremonies and other rituals for nurses. Burke and Matsumoto (1999) suggest specific ways in which a chaplain can be a supportive resource for staff. These ideas, presented in Box 8-1, summarize the various roles that chaplains fulfill.

Clergy

In one study, over 60 percent of hospitalized patients identified a clergyperson in the community whom they could reach if they wished (VandeCreek & Gibson, cited in VandeCreek, 1997). Clients (or one of

---

Box 8-1. How the Chaplain Can Be a Supportive Resource

Creator of Meaning: Chaplains can assist nurses in making sense of suffering, life, and death. They can help nurses to consider their own spiritual needs and wrestle with their own beliefs.

Trustworthy Listener: Chaplains can compassionately hear the stories and concerns of nurses without "taking sides."

Pastor Away from Home: Chaplains can minister to nurses when they don't have a minister or don't feel comfortable discussing their work with their own. Chaplains sometimes perform marriage ceremonies for nurses, or give them marital or grief counseling.

Calming Presence: Chaplains can provide comfort to nurses amidst emotionally stressful situations. For example, when nurses have to present bad news or conduct a family conference, the chaplain's presence can be calming.

Fellow Sojourner in the Land of Bereavement: Chaplains can help nurses to build and use supportive resources for coping with grief.

Generator of Ethical Concerns: Chaplains, because of their knowledge of ethics and religious principles, can assist nurses in identifying and understanding ethical concerns.

Educator: Chaplains can educate nurses about communicating with clients and about appreciating their spirituality.

Source: Burke, S. S., & Matsumoto, A. R. (1999). Pastoral care for perinatal and neonatal health care providers. *JOGNN: Journal of Obstetric, Gynecologic, & Neonatal Nursing, 28*(2), 137–141.

their family members) often inform their clergy of their health circumstances and needs. Some may not, however, because they may be too embarrassed or may believe their situation does not warrant contact. Thus, a client may express to the nurse a desire to see clergy, or the nurse may introduce the idea of a clergy referral. Either way, nurses have opportunities to collaborate with clergy in provision of spiritual care.

Practices vary with regard to the process for making a clergy referral. Chaplains working at health care institutions may want to act as an intermediary between the nurse and the clergy; they sometimes prefer to make the contact so that they can brief the clergy about the concerns of the client (VandeCreek, 1997). Furthermore, just as a primary care physician makes the referral for a client to a medical specialist, institutional policy may stipulate that chaplains make referrals to clergy. Nurses should be aware of any such policy and be sensitive to the practice preferred by the chaplains who serve their health care institution. In some institutions, however, the nurse may initiate a referral and/or make the contact with the client's clergy.

Clergy training is highly variable, not only in terms of theology, but also in degree of preparation for ministry. While some clergy will have earned graduate degrees in religious ministry, others may not have a college diploma. Even for those clergy who have received specialized education in their field, this education may not have included any study or practicum in how to care for persons with a health challenge. Some religious traditions utilize only lay ministers, or individuals who volunteer to minister to a congregation while continuing to work at a job.

This lack of specialized training for addressing the spiritual or religious concerns of the ill may explain why Spilka, Spangler, and Nelson (1983) observed complaints clients had about clergy and chaplains. They found the most common complaint was that these professionals "did nothing." Other complaints that clients expressed related to their perception of clergy and chaplains as insensitive, uncomfortable, and unable to communicate. It is such observations that apparently contributed to Taylor and Amenta's (1994) anecdotal evidence that some nurses will contact their own clergy to assist with their client's spiritual concerns when they dislike or are unable to contact the chaplain.

Parish Nurses

When a nurse cares for a client who is a member of a religious community that is served by a parish nurse, this parish nurse can be another resource for spiritual nurture. Parish nurses are registered nurses with special training who provide holistic care to members of a religious congregation. These nurses recognize and make the most of the link between faith and health. They collaborate with the minister(s) and staff of a congregation to promote health and prevent disease among the congregants. The roles of parish nurses are those of health educator, personal health counselor, volunteer coordinator, advocate and facilitator, role model, and referral agent or community liaison (Bay, 1997; Schank, Weis, & Matheus, 1996; Solari-Twadell & Westberg, 1991).

Modern parish nursing began in the 1980s in the Chicago area and has grown rapidly since. Parish nurses can be found in at least 48 states and 4 international locations (i.e., South Korea, Taiwan, Canada, and Australia [where they are called "faith community nurses"]). Over 2,500 nurses have completed a basic parish nurse program (personal communication, Ann Solari-Twadell, Director, International Parish Nurse Resource Center, May 23, 2000). While some parish nurses volunteer their services, others are hired by a congregation (Bay, 1997). Often, a hospital contracts with the congregation for the nurse's services. Some parish nurses may serve more than one congregation. These nurses may work full time or as few as 10 hours per week (Schank et al., 1996).

Parish nurses intend to complement the care provided by other members of the health care team. They do not duplicate the services of home health care nurses or public health nurses. They do not perform invasive procedures or administer medications (Schank et al., 1996). From studying clients who received parish nursing care, Rydholm (1997) found that half of concerns parish nurses address were of a physical nature, while the other half were of a "spiritual–psychosocial" nature (e.g., unresolved feelings, isolation, interpersonal tensions, caregiver stresses). Understanding the various roles of parish nurses (outlined in Box 8-2) will inform nurses as to what situations would benefit from referral to a parish nurse.

Although the educational backgrounds of parish nurses vary, all programs of study include instruction in spiritual caregiving. Some have received a master's degree or postbaccalaureate certificate, while others may have prepared through an extensive continuing education program in parish nursing.

Parish nurses know their parishioners intimately. Hence, they know the needs of clients' families and have insights about how compliant a client will be with medical treatments. To discuss a client case or make a referral, the nurse may need to contact the parish's office to get the contact

---

Box 8-2 Roles of the Parish Nurse

Health Educator: E.g., provides reading materials or lectures to the congregation on health-related topics (e.g., home safety, cancer prevention)

Personal Health Counselor: E.g., offers blood pressure measurement at the church/temple, and then advises congregants about how to better manage their blood pressure

Volunteer Coordinator: E.g., trains and manages volunteers to feed the hungry or visit the sick

Community Liaison/Referral Agent: E.g., connects congregants with community resources (e.g., agencies, information, people)

Role Model: E.g., serves as an example for how to eat and live healthfully, illustrates commitment to the congregation by attending services weekly

Advocate/Facilitator: E.g., organizes support groups, advocates for the marginalized members of the congregation

---

information for the parish nurse. Once the contact is established, the referring nurse can share with the parish nurse information about the client's current health situation and spiritual concerns.

Referrals to a parish nurse are especially warranted when the client has health concerns that have an impact on religious practices. Other situations that may indicate the need to refer include when the client lacks medical insurance and financial means for health care. The parish nurse can recruit resources to assist these economically needy parishioners. Referral to a parish nurse may be beneficial also when a client has poor social support. The parish nurse can recruit volunteers from the congregation to help. Also, when clients have spiritual issues they want to discuss with someone other than their clergy (e.g., a female patient whose minister is male who wants to talk with another woman, or patients who are embarrassed to talk with their clergy about their health problem), a referral to a parish nurse is appropriate. An interview with a parish nurse (see Box 8-3) offers an inside view of one nurse's experience in this area of nursing.

Box 8-3. One Nurse's Story: Interview with a Parish Nurse

A parish nurse for over a decade, Lou-Anne Keith, RN, MSN, NP-C, is employed by the Anaheim United Methodist Church in Anaheim, California.

Why did you choose this work?

I see my nursing as a ministry. I wanted to be able to integrate my nursing practice with my religious faith in a very intentional way.

What preparation did you obtain to become a parish nurse?

As a BSN student, I did an internship with a nurse who coordinated health ministries for a community hospital. During this internship, I participated in a one-day course that introduced the concepts of health ministries to me. Later, I attended a couple of the Health Ministries Association conferences. Most recently, I completed a 50-unit graduate program in parish nursing. This academic program allowed me to take three theology classes, a ministry class, electives, plus a unit of CPE. I think every parish nurse should have CPE.

How much do you work? And who pays you?

I am paid by the church to work 10 hours per week. The church also has a budget for health ministries. I spend this allowance for things like literature to hand out, maintaining a health supplies closet, wheelchairs, materials and lecturers for classes, and my own professional development.

Describe some of your activities.

I teach a weekly Bible class to help the congregation understand that if the spirit is broken, the body—and the emotions—are affected.

I confer with the ministers to assess what is going on healthwise for members of the congregation.

I also assess what is going on in the lives of the ministers.

I visit hospitalized members, or those who are sick at home.

I make phone calls to those who have asked for information or requested help.

I make contacts with community resources to plan health fairs or other events that I plan for the church.

(continues)

Box 8-3. One Nurse's Story: Interview with a Parish Nurse (continued)

I write notes to those who are ill or are grieving.

I talk with members about their health challenges. For example, I had a member recently who was going to have surgery on both her feet, had two school-aged kids, a two-story house, and a small bathroom that you couldn't push a wheelchair into. I strategized and helped educate her about how she could manage this problem.

When a member has a new baby, I make a stuffed animal and take it to the home and do a new baby assessment. Before the baby is born, I send the member a packet with information and a message from the pastor.

I am currently planning a series of classes for the youth in the church. I am assessing what topics would interest them. Then, during the classes, I'll recruit them to help me with the health fair I am planning.

I pray with and for members who are having health-related difficulties.

With whom do you collaborate?

Medical social workers and discharge planners. And nurses at the bedside. I also collaborate occasionally with physicians and hospice professionals. Of course, I work closely with the clergy. And I often collaborate with volunteer agency personnel (e.g., National Alliance for the Mentally Ill local chapter) and public health nurses when I organize a health fair, flu shots, or instructional session for the church.

What do you like most about your work?

I love teaching self-care. And the feeling of working together with God and the patient to promote health.

Spiritual Mentors

Spiritual mentors, or "spiritual directors" as they are typically called in Christian traditions, are people who assist others to develop spiritually. Spiritual directors are "holy listeners" (Guenther, 1992). For centuries, laypersons and clergy alike have adopted the habit of regularly meeting with a spiritual mentor. This is a practice that crosses many religious traditions. For individuals desiring spiritual discipline, regular visits (e.g., every 4 to 6 weeks) with a spiritual mentor are recommended. Times of crisis may provoke more frequent meetings.

Ideally, spiritual mentoring is offered by an individual trained specifically in spiritual direction. Often, spiritual mentors are religious professionals. Spiritual mentors may have received their preparation for providing spiritual direction from either a seminary or a program affiliated with a religious retreat center. Whereas some mentors (or their employers) will request pay, others offer their direction as a free gift to the client. Although a mentor and a mentee do not need to share the same religious orientation, it is necessary for mentees to be comfortable relating intimate matters of the soul and open to learning from the mentor. Thus, a director who is of the same gender and from a similar religious tradition is sometimes recommended (Leech, 1980).

Spiritual mentors and mentees generally devote their meetings to topics pertaining to the mentee's spiritual experience. Persons experiencing a health-related life transition or problem may find that exploring the spiritual dimension of their health with a spiritual mentor will help them to identify, understand, and resolve spiritual concerns. For example, a spiritual mentor can help an individual to understand how God is present in that challenge. Or a mentor may help a mentee living with physical pain to learn how to pray or meditate while in pain. Or a mentor may assist someone to make sense of his or her suffering, or to identify comforting religious beliefs to ease suffering. A spiritual mentor can not only encourage and comfort but also challenge one to strive for increased spiritual awareness and discipline.

It is highly unlikely that a nurse would make a referral to a spiritual director, unless the client identifies a director who has been helpful in the past. However, because health challenges often precipitate an awareness of spiritual need, the nurse can suggest to clients that a spiritual director might be helpful. Nurses can identify for clients the religious retreat centers or organizations (found in a telephone directory) in their area that offer spiritual direction and encourage clients to seek a director who is a good match for them.

Folk Healers

Across cultures of the world, especially where localized religions exist, healing of physical and mental ills is often sought from laypersons who are believed to have healing abilities. These "folk" healers (e.g., Haitian

priests and priestesses, Native American medicine men, Mexican curanderos, Russian shamans) typically use techniques distinct from Western
medicine such as rituals, divination, and native herbs and other natural
materials to promote health. Although education for folk healing has been
institutionalized in a few places, most folk healers receive their training
from apprenticeships, personal study, and experience.

Friends and Family

Although they are not trained as specialists in spiritual care, it is appropriate to remember who it is that clients prefer to have as a spiritual
resource person. Research findings indicate that clients often identify
friends and family as persons from whom they want spiritual nurture
(Highfield, 1992; Reed, 1991; Sodestrom, 1987). Friends and family
members can serve as supportive companions for those with health challenges. They can accompany. They can be empathic. They can share
comforting spiritual thoughts. They can pray. They can read or sing
inspiriting words. They can share a healing ritual. The history that friends
and family have with the client deepens the meaning to the spiritual care
that they give, sometimes unknowingly. When the help of spiritually supportive family and friends is available for a client, nurses can support the
client by assisting these individuals in their caregiving. For example, the
nurse can provide spiritually comforting materials for a friend to read to
the client who is feeling too sick to read. The nurse can serve as a role
model by demonstrating how to remain with a loved one who is in pain.
And nurses can encourage open dialogue about spiritual matters.

NURSING IMPLICATIONS

Collaborating with Spiritual Care Professionals

Effective collaboration between nurses and experts in spiritual caregiving
benefits client care and supports professional relationships. Research indicates that nurses generally value the services of chaplains and clergy, but
their rates for making referrals vary and can be low (Taylor & Amenta,
1994; Kristeller, Sheedy Zumbrun, & Schilling, 1999; Scott et al., 1994).
To encourage greater utilization of the expertise of spiritual care specialists, several suggestions will be offered. However, it is necessary to first
discuss when it is appropriate to make a referral to such a specialist.

Criteria for Initiating Referral

Not all clients have spiritual needs requiring assistance. Not all spiritual needs requiring assistance necessitate a referral. There are several situations, however, when the involvement of a spiritual care specialist should be mandatory. These include when:

- A client requests the service of an expert.
- A client's spiritual needs are complex, requiring knowledge and skills beyond those of the generalist nurse.
- A client's spiritual needs, if unmet, can threaten life (e.g., spiritual distress that could contribute to suicide, or hopelessness that could cause a premature death).

Other situations, however, also warrant referrals. When a spiritual need requires more emotional energy or time than a nurse has, others who have these resources should become involved in caring for the client. Or a client may prefer to discuss a religious concern with someone who shares the same religious tradition; if the nurse is of a different spiritual perspective, a specialist of the client's religious tradition should be called.

Although chaplains and clergy may offer their services 24 hours each day ("on call"), the nurse should consider the timing of a request for a patient visit. For example, these professionals should not be awakened to visit a client who has already died and had the relatives leave. A Roman Catholic patient near death who has already received the Sacrament of the Sick does not need to receive it again at the time of death (see Chapter 10). A concern that can be just as easily attended to during normal working hours should not be used to awaken a chaplain or clergyperson. Other routine pastoral care services that are best dealt with during business hours include responding to requests for communion, making general pastoral visits providing counseling, and offering religious materials.

The nurse may wonder which spiritual care expert to consult to assist a client. Typically, the client will have a preference. However, understanding the backgrounds and roles of these various experts can help guide the nurse to make an appropriate referral. For example, clients may recognize the need for someone to assist them with a spiritual need but may refuse to see a member of the clergy. The nurse can then suggest alternative specialists and query clients as to their preference. It is also possible that a client may want to meet with a clergyperson without having any religious affiliation or a prior relationship with a clergyperson. The nurse can then ask a chaplain to assess the client to determine which religious tradition matches the client's beliefs and identify a clergyperson to care for the client. If the chaplain is a clergyperson, as most are, the chaplain may address such client needs.

Guidelines for Enhancing the Collaborative Process

Ideal collaborative care entails discussing the client's situation with the spiritual care expert both before and after a visit. (This applies mostly to chaplain and clergy visitation of clients.) Before a visit, the nurse can inform the expert of pertinent information and answer questions the expert may have. After the visit, the expert may have valuable assessment information or ideas to enhance the nurse's plan for spiritual care. When nurses involve specialists in the assessment and plan of care, they improve the quality of spiritual care delivered and eliminate redundant assessments.

During the chaplain or clergy visit with a client, interruptions should be avoided. The nurse strives to coordinate and schedule care so as to minimize unnecessary intrusions. A notice can be placed on the client's door to encourage others to respect this sacred time, for example, "Pastoral Ministry Taking Place—Please Do Not Disturb."

The nurse can assist spiritual care specialists in other ways as well. Some specialists may benefit from a nurse's sensitivity to the shock or discomfort that the specialist may experience in response to interacting with the client. Although many specialists are prepared to encounter serious illness, pain, and other forms of suffering, as well as catheters, intravenous lines, and other medical equipment, others may need support. Even experienced specialists may feel uncomfortable around a client whose condition is grave. If the specialist and the client have previously had a close relationship, the specialist may be personally shocked by the client's situation and thus may benefit from support of an informational or emotional nature from the nurse.

A nurse can offer the specialist a brief orientation about the patient's illness, treatment, and environment in such a manner that prepares the specialist for the emotional challenge of meeting the client. Sights (e.g., disfigurement), smells (e.g., necrotic tissue), and sounds (e.g., ventilator machine) that may be difficult to be around can be explained to the specialist beforehand. For example, the nurse may offer a sensitive statement like, "It can be hard for me to look into the eyes of patients like this whose faces are so disfigured. You may find it is the same way for you."

If a nurse senses that a spiritual care expert ministering to a client is uncomfortable, the nurse may be able to share suggestions with that specialist about how to attend to the client. For instance, a specialist who has never cared for a comatose patient will likely appreciate a few encouraging tips from a nurse about how to communicate or be present. Or a specialist visiting an intensive care unit for the first time may welcome a nurse's explaining the client's situation and medical paraphernalia briefly.

When collaborating with a specialist, the nurse should use appropriate language, considering that the specialist likely has not learned much medical jargon. To illustrate, a nurse might say something like this to a specialist about to visit a colonectomy patient: "Our client had part of his gut removed three days ago, so you may see, hear, or smell stool that is collecting in a plastic bag on his abdomen. This bag, called a colostomy bag, is typically upsetting initially for clients. I think he may benefit from discussing with you how his physically damaged body deters his spirit." Likewise, if a specialist uses language or theological concepts that are unfamiliar to the nurse, the nurse should not hesitate to request an explanation.

It is also possible that the client may be emotionally raw after a visit from a spiritual care expert. Discussing one's deeply personal spiritual concerns can bring tears, quiet withdrawal, and a range of emotions to the surface. These reactions are not bad; in fact, they are likely to be ultimately healing. If such emotions are observed after a spiritual care expert leaves a client, the patient may desire support from the nurse—or may want to be left alone. Either way, it is probably incorrect to conclude that the expert disturbed the client. Rather, it would be appropriate for the nurse to follow up with the client and assess how to be supportive during this tender time. The nurse may learn that it would be best to minimize activity in the client's room so that quiet reflection or prayer can occur, or the nurse may learn the client wishes to talk further about issues that the specialist raised.

If a client is resistant to the nurse's recommendation of a referral to a spiritual care expert, the appropriate response most often is not to drop the idea. Instead, the nurse may gently query the client as to what contributes to the resistance (e.g., "I'm sensing you don't feel comfortable with my suggestion; can you help me understand why?"). Allowing clients to discuss their resistance may help them to overcome it. Examples of reasons for this resistance may include:

- Denial that there is a spiritual need
- Discomfort with the idea of disclosing such intimate personal experience (e.g., embarrassed by a "sin," guilt about thinking doubtfully)
- A previous negative encounter with a spiritual care expert

Clergy, and even chaplains, can sometimes trigger negative associations for a client who has had a negative encounter with a spiritual care expert or religious institution in the past. A client who refuses to see a spiritual care expert may be receptive to a nurse who is able to address spiritual concerns with sensitivity.

Although time constraints sometimes prevent it, gaining a client's permission before making a referral is recommended. A likely time to gain a client's permission is at the conclusion of a spiritual assessment. A nurse might ask, for example, "I am sensing that you have a lot of questions about why suffering exists. Is there an expert you'd like me to have in to discuss these perplexities with you?" As with physicians who may consult a specialist without informing a patient, nurses also often call in a chaplain without inquiring if the patient desires this visit. Clients, however, will likely be more receptive to a spiritual care expert if they have approved the referral.

When the client does refuse to see a spiritual care expert, the nurse must respect the client's wishes. However, a nurse may still consult with an expert. While discussing the client's care, it is ethical to refrain from divulging any information that would betray the client's identity. There may be other circumstances in which the nurse should not divulge confidential client information. Nurses must remember that clients may not want their nurses to share medical information with their spiritual care expert, if this individual is not a member of the health care team. Nurses should be sensitive to this and respectful of clients' desires for privacy.

Collaboration between nurses and spiritual care professionals allows for the provision of effective spiritual care for clients. Although nurses frequently make referrals to chaplains, nurses can enhance patient care by considering how they can collaborate with other spiritual care professionals and take an active role in helping these professionals to provide spiritual care. The case presented in Box 8-4 illustrates how one nurse collaborated with others to provide spiritual care.

Box 8-4. Case Study: Collaborating with a Spiritual Care Specialist

Mr. Lee, a 47-year-old Chinese American biologist, was diagnosed five years ago with lung cancer. Mr. Lee and his wife of 25 years have two college-aged children. When it was recognized that he did not have more than six months to live, Mr. Lee agreed to receive hospice care in his home. Susan Adamson, RN, was the primary nurse assigned to care for Mr. Lee.

When conducting her initial assessment, Nurse Adamson included questions to help her assess for Mr. Lee's spiritual needs and learned that Mr. Lee did not consider himself religious. She learned, however, that throughout his childhood, Mr. Lee visited a Buddhist temple weekly with his parents. She sensed a wistfulness as he talked about memories of these temple visits and hearing his mother pray. She also learned that the spiritual values most important to him were harmonious relationships with family and with nature. That is, he firmly believed that children ought to respect their elders, and he maintained a deep respect as a biologist for the mystery and beauty in nature. He mentioned, however, that he felt disillusioned with nature now that he was observing how it bred cancer within his body. He was also troubled by his children's diminished respect for him and his wife.

Nurse Adamson recognized that Mr. Lee's need to give and receive love (e.g., from children) and the need to reconstruct hope and meaning (e.g., in nature or whatever he perceived as divine) were spiritual needs. She also intuited that Mr. Lee would like to revisit the religiosity of his mother.

Nurse Adamson informed Mr. Lee, per hospice policy, about the automatic referral she would make for him to the hospice's chaplain. When he learned of the referral, he refused the offer of a chaplain, stating, "Oh, I'm not a Christian; I'm not even religious; I don't want to see a chaplain!" Even when the nurse clarified that chaplains are interested in supporting clients spiritually, regardless of religiosity, Mr. Lee refused the care.

(continues)

> **Box 8-4. Case Study: Collaborating with a Spiritual Care Specialist** *(continued)*

Nurse Adamson, having identified the existence of spiritual needs but unable to secure Mr. Lee's permission to allow a chaplain to address them, had to creatively plan spiritual care for her client. First, she consulted with the hospice chaplain. After describing the data she collected during her spiritual assessment of Mr. Lee (without confiding his identity), she was able to have the chaplain help her to pinpoint Mr. Lee's most serious spiritual needs and to identify spiritual care professionals who might help. These included a Chinese Buddhist volunteer chaplain at a nearby hospital and a monk who functioned as a spiritual mentor at a Buddhist temple in a city 25 miles away. The chaplain also suggested how Nurse Adamson could address Mr. Lee's need for love, hope, and meaning.

Although Mr. Lee was excited about the idea of having weekly conversations with the monk, his health allowed him the luxury of only four visits. However, he was able to continue his dialogue with this monk over the Internet until his mind became fuzzy from opioids. Along with this spiritual care came compassion from his wife, neighbors, former colleagues, and nurses. By the end of his life, he came to enjoy an increased awareness and experience of love. He also had a restored appreciation for nature and his place in it.

Because of the spiritual peace his children observed during his dying, they demonstrated increased respect for him. Mr. Lee beamed one evening when his son asked, "Dad, I'm so impressed! How come you are so calm and peaceful even though you're dying?" Mr. Lee died peacefully two days later.

KEY POINTS

- Nurses typically are generalists in spiritual caregiving, while those professionals who have received advanced education in spiritual counseling are the experts.

- Spiritual care experts include chaplains, clergy, spiritual directors, parish nurses, and folk healers. Clients, however, often prefer to have their own family or friends help them with spiritual needs.
- Nurses collaborate with spiritual care experts in a number of ways, including:
  - Discussing the client's care with the expert before and after the expert serves the client
  - Being respectful of a client's need for privacy regarding spiritual matters
  - Assisting experts who are uncomfortable with ministering to sick persons or in health care environments
  - Not avoiding a spiritual need requiring a referral or consultation even when a client resists it
  - Including clients in the referral process
  - Considering the expert's personal needs while determining when to contact the expert

LOOK WITHIN TO LEARN

1. What experiences have you had with spiritual care experts? Are your impressions of them positive or negative? How might these perceptions influence to whom and how you would make a referral?

2. If you were a patient experiencing a spiritual need, who would you want to have help you? Why?

3. If you were a patient with a spiritual need, how would you want your nurse to introduce the idea of making a referral for you to a spiritual care expert?

4. When making a referral, what client information do you believe would be helpful or appropriate to offer to the spiritual care expert?

REFERENCES

Bold print indicates those that are most recommended.

Association of Professional Chaplains. (May, 2000). Available on-line: *http://www.professionalchaplains.org.*

Bay, M. J. (1997). Healing partners: The oncology nurse and the parish nurse. *Seminars in Oncology Nursing, 13,* 275–278.

Burke, S. S., & Matsumoto, A. R. (1999). Pastoral care for perinatal and neonatal health care providers. *JOGNN: Journal of Obstetric, Gynecologic, & Neonatal Nursing, 28*(2), 137–141.

Gallup, G. H., Jr. (1996). *Religion in America.* Princeton, NJ: Princeton Religion Research Center.

Guenther, M. (1992). *Holy listening: The art of spiritual direction.* Boston: Cowley.

Highfield, M. F. (1992). Spiritual health of oncology patients: Nurse and patient perspectives. *Cancer Nursing, 15,* 1–8.

Highfield, M. E. F., Taylor, E. J., & Amenta, M. (2000). Preparation to care: The spiritual care education of oncology and hospice nurses. *Journal of Hospice and Palliative Care, 2*(2), 53–63.

Kristeller, J. L., Sheedy Zumbrun, C., & Schilling, R. F. (1999). "I would if I could": How oncology nurses address spiritual distress in cancer patients. *Psycho-Oncology, 8,* 451–458.

Leech, K. (1980). *Soul friend: The practice of Christian spirituality.* San Francisco: Harper & Row.

McSherry, W. (1998). Nurses' perceptions of spirituality and spiritual care. *Nursing Standard, 13*(4), 36–40.

Reed, P. G. (1991). Preferences for spiritually related nursing interventions among terminally ill and nonterminally ill hospitalized adults and well adults. *Applied Nursing Research, 4,* 122–128.

Rydholm, L. (1997). Patient-focused care in parish nursing. *Holistic Nursing Practice, 11*(3), 47–60.

Schank, M. J., Weis, D., & Matheus, R. (1996). Parish nursing: Ministry of healing. *Geriatric Nursing, 17*(1), 11–13.

Scott, M. S., Grzybowski, M., & Webb, S. (1994). Perceptions and practices of registered nurses regarding pastoral care and the spiritual need of hospital patients. *Journal of Pastoral Care, 48,* 171–179.

Sodestrom, K. E., & Martinson, I. M. (1987). Patients' spiritual coping strategies: A study of nurse and patient perspectives. *Oncology Nursing Forum, 14,* 41–45.

Solari-Twadell, A., & Westberg, G. (1991). Body, mind, and soul: The parish nurse offers physical, emotional, and spiritual care. *Health Progress,* 24–28.

Spilka, B., Spangler, J. D., & Nelson, C. B. (1983). Spiritual support in life threatening illness. *Jouronal of Religion and Health, 22*(2), 98–104.

Taylor, E. J., Highfield, M. F., & Amenta, M. O. (1999). Predictors of oncology and hospice nurses spiritual care perspectives and practices. *Applied Nursing Research, 12*(1), 30–37.

Taylor, E. J., Highfield, M., & Amenta, M. (1994). Attitudes and beliefs regarding spiritual care: A survey of cancer nurses. *Cancer Nursing, 17*(6), 479–487.

Taylor, E. J., & Amenta, M. O. (1994). Cancer Nurses' Perspectives on Spiritual Care: Implications for Pastoral Care. *Journal of Pastoral Care, 48*(3), 259–265.

VandeCreek, L. (1997). Collaboration between nurses and chaplains for spiritual caregiving. *Seminars in Oncology Nursing, 13,* 279–280.

VandeCreek, L., Carl, D., & Parker, D. (1998). The role of nonparish clergy in the mental health system. In H. Koenig (Ed.), *Handbook of religion and mental health* (pp. 337–348). San Diego, CA: Academic Press.

Part III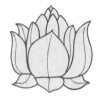

Promoting Spiritual Health

9

Supporting Spiritual Health Through Ritual

Weddings, funerals, nurses' pinning ceremonies, and baptisms are examples of rituals or ceremonial acts that are regularly performed in a set manner. Rituals also include activities such as making pancakes every Sunday morning, visiting a loved one's grave, or marking an anniversary with a special gift. Regardless of the form they take, rituals provide a way for people to make meaning of their life experiences. Some rituals help people to reconnect with their spirituality and thus support spiritual health. Prayer and meditation, for example, are rituals that can promote spirituality. This chapter will explore how nurses can facilitate client use of ritual in order to promote spiritual health.

Imber-Black and Roberts (1993) propose a broad definition for rituals as "symbolic acts that . . . are 'held' together by a guiding metaphor" (p. 8). Rituals are not restricted to groups; one person alone can create and implement a ritual. A client, for example, might engage in a solitary daily ritual of devotional reading and prayer to commune with God.

Hammerschlag and Silverman (1997) distinguish ceremony from ritual. While rituals are actions that are repeated, occasionally without meaning or reason, ceremonies are a type of ritual that is performed in order to commemorate special events that occur once in a while. Nurses participate often in health care rituals and sometimes in ceremonies. Frequent measurement of vital signs, daily baths, grand rounds, and many other routinized aspects of health care are rituals. While many health care rituals address medical, physical, or even social needs, the purpose of some may no longer be justifiable (e.g., bathing infants every day). A ceremonial ritual that nurses sometimes participate in is a memorial service for a client for whom they have provided care.

COMPONENTS OF RITUAL

Imber-Black and Roberts (1993) reviewed various aspects of ritual, including repetition, special or stylized behavior, order, an evocative presentation, and a social dimension. These multiple aspects of ritual are illustrated in the pinning ceremony for graduating nursing students. This ceremony is repeated yearly in a nursing school to mark entry of students into the profession of nursing. Graduating students are not merely saying or thinking "I am now a professional nurse," but behaving in a way that signifies change from student to professional. A school pin is affixed by a special person. Pinning ceremonies, like most rituals, follow an order or agenda (e.g., a welcome message, special music, speeches, pinning, recitation of the Pledge, dismissal). Uniforms or dressy clothing, flowers and other decorations, and music illustrate the evocative presentation of ritual that serves to focus attention at a pinning. The social dimension is represented by friends and family who attend a pinning.

FUNCTIONS OF RITUAL

Ultimately, rituals function to "separate the ordinary from the extraordinary" (Hammerschlag & Silverman, 1997). A ritual is created to bring about a good outcome or to make something special. Because rituals reflect people's deepest thoughts and feelings, they often are overtly spiritual or make reference to spiritual beings. Rituals also assist people facing challenge to manage change in a symbolic way (Froggatt, 1997; Acterberg, Dossey, & Kolkmeier, 1994). Rituals support people spiritually by enabling them to relate, change, heal, believe, and celebrate (Imber-Black & Roberts, 1993):

- Rituals allow people to shape, express, and maintain relationships. A funeral, for example, helps a family who has lost a member to feel supported by friends. The ritual of a mealtime not only helps families or friends to stay connected, but expresses how the individuals relate to each (e.g., who determines who says the "grace" can indicate who is the religious patriarch for the group).
- Rituals enable change by aiding individuals to make and mark transitions in life. Rituals make the change feel manageable and safe. As a "coming of age" ritual marks the transition from child to adult, it enacts a change that cannot occur by simply making the statement, "I am an adult now!" Rituals can help clients to mark transitions like menopause, the end of treatments, or a change in health status.
- Rituals enable healing by helping people to recover from betrayals, traumas, or losses. A survivor of rape or abuse, for example, may find healing in a ritual designed to acknowledge and bury bitterness, helplessness, or hopelessness. A client who suffers from a physical or social disability may find healing in a ritual that transforms anger about the disability to energy for helping others.
- Rituals allow individuals to express their beliefs and make sense of them. The rituals inherent in a religious worship service, for an obvious example, express the beliefs of that religion.
- Rituals allow people to celebrate by helping them to affirm deep joys and honor life with festivity (e.g., Thanksgiving dinners, baby dedications or naming ceremonies, and family reunions). Most rituals involve a sense of appreciation for life and connectedness to others.

Ritual is often linked with healing (Achterberg, Dossey, & Kolkmeier, 1994; Hammerschlag & Silverman, 1997). Achterberg and colleagues identified several measurable health benefits that rituals have been found to influence. Positive outcomes of ritual include decreased levels of anxiety, depression, and feelings of helplessness, and an increased sense of social support, self-acceptance, and self-worth.

THE RITUAL OF PRAYER

An encyclopedia of religion defines *prayer* simply as "human communication with divine and spiritual entities" (Gill, 1987, p. 489). While some argue that not all people in all cultures and religions pray, others posit that it is a universal phenomenon (Wierzbicka, 1994). Ulanov and Ulanov (1982), for example, proposed that all do pray:

> *People pray whether or not they call it prayer. We pray every time we ask*
> *for help, understanding, or strength, in or out of religion . . . who and what*
> *we are speak out of us. . . . To pray is to listen to and hear this self who is*
> *speaking. (p. 1)*

Because prayer is often practiced outside of religious contexts by nonreligious persons, it is included here as a spiritual ritual rather than a religious practice. Aspects of prayer that emerge within religious contexts are presented in Chapter 10.

Dossey described prayer as intention plus love. That is, prayer is a loving wish or thought for oneself or another. Dossey, as do most who define prayer, acknowledges that prayer is often communicated with "the Absolute," a term useful for describing that ultimate power in which any person praying might believe. Prayer is not an invocation of positive or negative forms of magic, nor does it represent an unloving intent ("Conversations," 1999). Dossey believes that a nurse who harbors negative thoughts towards a client can be harmful to that client. Remembering that prayer involves a desire for connection with a divine entity rather than a summons for magical power on behalf of the person petitioning will help guide nurses to an appropriate attitude for prayer. The common prayerful phrase "God's will be done" (rather than "My will be done") is also indicative of an appropriate approach to prayer.

Survey research completed during the past several decades has consistently found that about 90 percent of Americans report a belief in prayer (Poloma & Gallup, 1991). Furthermore, of those who engage in prayer, 95 percent indicate that they believe their prayers have "been answered," and 86 percent believe that their prayers have made them a "better person" (Gallup, 1996). Research suggests that persons who are experiencing physiologic or mental health challenges may use prayer even more (see pp. 206–207). Considering these findings, it is not surprising that many clients state that they would like their physician to pray with them (i.e., 67 percent and 48 percent of Oyama & Koenig's (1998) and King & Bushwick's (1994) study participants, respectively). Although no published research reports as yet suggest what percentage of clients would want their nurses to pray with or for them, evidence indicates that clients value the ability of the nurse to show sensitivity to their spirituality and the spiritual coping strategies they employ (see Chapter 2). Because of the intimate and caring nature of the nurse–client relationship, a client may feel more comfortable praying with a nurse than with a physician. Close client contact is inherent in the practice of nursing. Nurses, therefore, are more likely to be available when a client experiences a need to share prayer.

Although some nurses may feel uncomfortable with the idea of praying overtly *with* a client, many report that they do pray privately *for* clients. To illustrate, 66 percent of 181 oncology nurses (Taylor, Amenta, & Highfield, 1995) and 53 percent of 571 critical care nurses (Rozanski, 1997) reported that they pray "often" or "very often" for their clients. Despite indicating frequent private prayer, however, nurses report that they rarely pray with clients (Taylor, Amenta, & Highfield, 1995; Rozanski, 1997; McRoberts, Sato, & Southwick, 2000).

Two studies have assessed nurses' use of complementary therapies, including prayer. Taylor and colleagues (1998) surveyed emergency department personnel (78 percent of whom were nurses) and found that 47 percent acknowledged recommending "prayer or spiritual practices" to their clients. Two-thirds of these respondents believed these practices to be very effective. King and colleagues' (King, Pettigrew, & Reed, 2000) survey of 467 Ohio nurses found that although 81 percent personally used prayer and rated it second as the most effective complementary therapy, only 30 percent reported using it with clients.

Types of Prayer

Poloma and Gallup (1991) observed that Americans engage in four types of prayer: meditative, colloquial, petitionary, and ritual. Meditative prayers involve maintaining a sense of openness toward the divine and are not dependent on thoughts and words. Colloquial or conversational prayers involve thinking or speaking spontaneously, as in conversation with the divine. Petitionary prayers are prayers of specific requests for divine help. Ritual prayers are prayers that are repeated, created by another, and often found in religious literature. Interestingly, in a study with a large sampling of healthy adults, these researchers found that meditative and colloquial prayers were significantly more associated with overall reports of spiritual well-being than were ritual and petitionary prayers. Others have distinguished different types of prayer by purpose, including to express lament, confess, intercede, praise or adore, express thanksgiving, and invoke or summon (Dossey, 1993).

Dossey (1993) highlighted the differences between the traditional, Western model of prayer and a "modern" model. In the traditional model, a conscious thought is conveyed to an external object of prayer (usually a higher power). The prayer is said in the present with the intent to change the future. In contrast, a modern model accepts that prayer is not limited by where or when it is experienced. Prayer may occur within an individual; it may be an inner experience of awareness of the divine within. Prayer also can occur without conscious thought; it may be preconscious or a dream prayer. Although Dossey distinguishes these two models, it is likely that many people accept parts of both of them.

Effects of Prayer

Research findings indicate that prayer may contribute to physical and emotional health. Many clients use prayer as a coping strategy, and many want their health care professional to pray with them.

Levin (1996) proposed a theoretical model that suggests four mechanisms that may explain why prayer brings about the healing effects that research observes. These mechanisms are either naturalistic (i.e., within the realm of nature) or supernatural (i.e., outside of nature and beyond human testing), combined with either locality (i.e., confined by space and time) or nonlocality (i.e., not limited to space and time as it is commonly understood). A local–naturalistic cause of healing by prayer, for example, could be explained by the effect of social support often experienced by those who pray or a psychoneuroimmunological response to faith. In contrast, a nonlocal–supernatural mechanism for healing could be explained by the intervening response of God, which is mysterious and ultimately beyond human examination.

Several researchers have compared the findings of several studies that test the effectiveness of prayer, intentionality, or other types of distance healing (Astin, Harkness, & Ernst, 2000; Dossey, 1993; Roberts, Ahmed, Hall, & Sargent, 2000; Targ, 1997). Dossey concluded that there is ample evidence to support belief that prayer physically heals and cures ill people and biological systems (e.g., fungi). Other reviews, however, conclude that evidence thus far is inconclusive, although promising. Roberts and Astin examined experimental studies of intercessory prayer (in contrast to other forms of distance healing which may be broader or different from prayer), and concluded that there is not enough evidence

yet to guide clinical practice. Astin and colleagues found only five intercessory prayer experiments to analyze, only two of which demonstrated a
significant positive effect.

These two landmark studies suggest that intercessory prayer may have
a significant effect on the physical health of the hospitalized client. Using a
double-blind experimental protocol, Byrd (1988) found a difference in certain medical outcomes among coronary care unit (CCU) patients who had
been prayed for by a group of "born again" Christians. The 192 recipients of
intercessory prayer were statistically more likely to have had fewer antibiotics and diuretics, and less intubation/ventilation than the 201 control
patients. Replicating this study, Harris and colleagues (1999) attempted to
address the methodological criticisms the Byrd experiment received and
still obtained similar results. These researchers observed significantly lower
overall adverse outcomes among CCU patients (n = 1,019).

Although experimental evidence of prayer's curative effect is inconclusive, there have been several correlational studies that demonstrate relationships between prayer and psychological health benefits. One of these
studies, conducted by nurse researchers (Meisenhelder & Chandler, 2000)
is presented in Box 9-1. Other research about health correlates of prayer
demonstrate that prayer is directly related to a sense of purpose among
healthy adults (Richards, 1991), is associated with less "current [psycho-
logical] distress" among coronary artery bypass graft (CABG) recipients
who prayed than among those who did not pray (Ai, Dunkle, Peterson, &
Bolling, 1998), improves self-esteem and lessens anxiety and depression
(O'Laoire, 1997), and is perceived as an effective coping strategy by clients
and their family caregivers (e.g., Stolley, Buckwalter, & Koenig, 1999).

**Box 9-1. Research Profile: Prayer and Health Outcomes
in Church Members**

Purpose: To measure the relationship between frequency of prayer
and various physical and mental health outcomes.

Methods: Data were collected with questionnaires mailed to members
of the Presbyterian Church, USA. The 1,025 respondents completed
the Medical Outcomes Study Short-form and one Likert item assessing frequency of prayer.

Main Findings: Frequency of prayer significantly correlated positively with poor physical function (r = 0.52), role function (r = 0. 21),

(continues)

Box 9-1. Research Profile: Prayer and Health Outcomes in Church Members *(continued)*

---

and bodily pain (r = 0.18), and better mental health (r = 0.28). People who prayed more frequently, therefore, were those who had poorer health and were older. Prayer appeared to have assisted these disadvantaged individuals by providing them with better mental health.

Nursing Implications: Although the researchers do not delineate clinical implications, their findings suggest that prayer may be a protective mechanism that fosters emotional health when religious persons face physical disease and aging. Nursing activities that support prayer may thus support mental health.

Source: Meisenhelder, J. B., & Chandler, E. N. (2000). Prayer and health outcomes in church members. *Alternative Therapies in Health and Medicine, 6*(4), 56–60.

Research findings indicate that people often use prayer to cope with their health concerns. Whether the health challenge is chronic pain (e.g., Ashby & Lenhart, 1994), cancer (e.g., Taylor, Outlaw, Bernardo, & Roy, 1999), AIDS (Carson, 1993), sickle cell anemia (Ohaeri, Shokunbi, Akinlade, & Dare, 1995), chronic renal disease (e.g., Sutton & Murphy, 1989), pregnancy (Levin, Lyons, & Larson, 1993), arthritis (Boisset & Fitzcharles, 1994), or an acute attack of cystitis (Webster & Brennan, 1995), clients use prayer to cope. Several studies also indicate that prayer is used by the elderly as they cope with the symptoms of aging and concerns about facing death (e.g., Bearon & Koenig, 1990). Prayer also has been identified by clients as a useful strategy for coping with diagnostic or therapeutic medical interventions such as a computed tomography scan (Peteet et al., 1992) and coronary artery bypass grafting (Saudia, Kinney, Brown, & Young-Ward, 1991).

Research findings indicate that faith and prayer may be a frequently used and highly valued strategy for coping. Several studies, for example, have found that participants rank as their first or second most important coping strategy "faith" and "prayer" (e.g., Sutton & Murphy, 1989). Other studies indicate that a majority of clients use faith and prayer to cope. Saudia and colleagues (1991), for example, found that 96 of 100 CABG patients reported prayer was used; 70 of these patients responded that prayer was "extremely helpful." Although most studies observe that at least half of participants report using prayer to cope, much variability exists among the studies regarding what percentage of respondents identified prayer as a coping strategy. In a frequently cited telephone survey study, 25 percent of 1,539 adults responded affirmatively when asked if prayer was used during the past year as a "medical therapy or treatment" (Eisenberg et al., 1993). The significant difference between Eisenberg's finding and other studies of those with illnesses who report higher usage of spiritual coping strategies may be explained by the seriousness of the health problem and hospitalization, which increases the frequency and importance of prayer as a coping strategy for people.

MEDITATION

Meditation is "the practice of focusing and concentrating one's attention and awareness while maintaining a passive attitude . . . [and is] a road to spiritual transformation" (Anselmo & Kolkmeier, 2000). May (1982), a psychiatrist well informed about various faith traditions, argued that meditation in its purest sense is one type of prayer experience. However, May recognized that contemporary meditation practices are often distinguishable from prayer by their lack of directedness toward a divine entity. Because many practice meditation regularly in a prescribed manner, it can also be considered a ritual.

After studying meditation in many different cultures and religions, Benson (1997) concluded that maintaining a passive, alert focus on meaningful thought was essential to attaining a "relaxation response." Benson proposed the following as steps in the practice of meditation. The nurse can easily teach these steps to a client directly or by providing written instructions.

- Select a brief, meaningful word or phrase (i.e., mantra) to repeat during the meditation. This phrase or word may be selected from sacred writings, a meaningful poem, ritual prayer, or some religious saying.
- Assume a comfortable position (an upright position is recommended).
- Close eyes (to minimize distraction and encourage focusing).
- Relax muscles (a simplified progressive muscle relaxation exercise may be helpful just prior to meditation).

- Become aware of breathing (a slow, rhythmic pattern will aid meditation).
- Maintain a passive attitude (i.e., when inner thoughts distract from the mantra, let them pass knowing you can think about them later, and return to the mantra).

While some meditational techniques involve repeating a mantra for a specified time, others suggest the mantra be contemplated in depth, allowing for personal applications to life. A mantra or centering prayer is often more helpful when it is constructed as an affirmation. "The Lord has mercy on me," for example, may be more helpful than "Have mercy on me, Lord." While some clients may prefer sitting still while meditating, others may benefit from combining this technique with physical movement. It is essential that the client determine the mantra, though the nurse may suggest options or help the client to reframe a chosen mantra as an affirmation.

NURSING IMPLICATIONS

Supporting Client Rituals

For many clients, meaningful ritual experiences already exist. The role of the nurse will be to assist in their continuation. A nurse may need to plan medications around a client's daily spiritual rituals or ensure quiet and privacy during prayer. A nurse may need to obtain ritualistic objects that the clients finds meaningful (e.g., rosary, prayer book, beads, candle) or prepare the client for the ritual (e.g, wash his hands, assist with dressing). The use of some ritual objects may be banned in some institutional settings (e.g., incense or an open flame). In these situations, the nurse becomes an advocate and negotiator, contacting the client's spiritual leader (via the chaplain, see Chapter 4) to identify alternative metaphors or methods.

The core of an effective ritual is the metaphor or symbol guiding the ritual. The metaphoric act of placing sacred oil on a client's forehead to represent a sacred balm or divine blessing, for example, is central to many healing rituals. Singing, scripture readings, and prayers that may be incorporated in a healing ritual are often incantations to prepare for this sacred experience. Such a ritual will be ineffective if the metaphor is inappropriate or meaningless to the client. Armstrong (1998) observed that the body informs a person as to whether the metaphor works; it works if the "spine tingles" or "goosebumps rise" or if it causes a deep breath or a stronger heartbeat. While this certainly may be true for many ritual experiences, it may not always apply. Spiritually mature individuals recognize that there are seasons in one's spiritual life. Just as there are peak experiences with intense emotional and sensational physical sequelae, there are also times when people sense a spiritual dullness, dryness, or "dark night of the soul" (as an early Christian mystic described it). The nurse reassures clients by helping them to recognize that strong feelings may or may not occur and that this is normal. A nurse may assist a client to determine if the ritual feels meaningless because the underlying metaphor is inappropriate or because the client is currently experiencing a spiritually dry season.

Those who find themselves unmoved by rituals may have beliefs that differ from those expressed in the messages of the ritual. If a genuine sense of joy is missing from a ritual, Imber-Black and Roberts (1993) contend, it is an indicator that some emotional work is needed. A lack of joy in a ritual may indicate a distressed relationship or a loss that needs to be talked about, resolved, and healed. When prayer, for example, seems ineffectual, unsatisfying, or boring, it may be attributable to a distressed relationship with the divine entity, an approach to prayer that has become threadbare, or a type of prayer that is mismatched with the personality or current circumstances. When nurses hear clients speak of useless rituals, they may encourage clients to explore what would effectively recreate the ritual.

Creating Rituals

Clients often need to mark a transition, grieve a loss, recognize a change, or celebrate life. Because ritual helps clients to attend to these needs, the nurse should encourage clients to perform personal rituals. Several points are important for nurses to remember as they assist clients with rituals.

When it is determined that a ritual might be an appropriate spiritual care intervention for a client, the nurse will need to introduce the idea of a ritual by discussing its value with the client. A nurse might say something like:

I am hearing you say "I want to get on with my life" but that it is difficult for you to do because of the way other people see you as disabled. You may find that creating a ritual to mark this change would be helpful, because rituals help us to bring into focus things like transitions. They can also help us to express how we think and feel and want to relate to others.

Creating a ritual may be a new experience for the client. Providing examples of how other clients have benefited from a healing ritual may encourage the client to consider developing an appropriate ritual.

It is essential that the client actively participate in planning most, if not all, of the ritual. Only the client knows what metaphors and aspects of ritual will meaningfully communicate the necessary message. Furthermore, much of the healing that comes from rituals occurs during the planning and preparation for the ritual. The client, therefore, must embrace the idea of creating of a ritual and play a key role in implementing it.

There are several areas to consider when planning a ceremonial ritual (Achterberg, Dossey, & Kolkmeier, 1994; Hammerschlag & Silverman, 1997; Imber-Black & Roberts, 1993):

- Planning for a ritual is based on a clear understanding of the ritual's purpose. What is it that the client wishes to have happen as a result? Is there a hidden agenda that needs to be addressed openly in the ritual?
- Pressures from others may influence how a client plans a ritual. Although a ritual needs to meet the needs of a client, the client may want to design the ritual so that other participants' needs are also met. A widower who wants to commemorate the first anniversary of his wife's death as a time to end mourning, for example, will likely consider expectations that his children and society have for bereaved individuals.
- Preparation for the ritual may involve shopping, inviting friends, cooking food, preparing special clothing or decorations, writing a poem or liturgy, or other activities. If clients are unable to do all the preparation, they can still determine the preparations needed and who will be responsible for them.
- The client should also determine who will and will not be invited to participate in or witness the ritual. Often, friends and family are important invitees, but health care professionals may also be meaningful participants. Clients who have requested that their clergyperson conduct a religious healing service often remark that they were comforted by the presence of their nurse at the ritual.
- The place where a ritual is performed holds symbolic meaning and needs to be carefully considered. It will, in essence, become a sacred space. Although they may select geographic locations known for sacredness or healing powers, clients can assign sacredness to any space, even a hospital room.

- The activities to be experienced during the ritual are salient aspects to consider. What will be the role of attendees? Will they silently support or actively participate? Hammerschlag and Silverman (1997) suggest that having a facilitator is helpful. Clients may select a representative from their spiritual community or a family patriarch/matriarch.
- Materials or "sacraments" to be used influence the atmosphere of a ceremony. Smelling incense, seeing flowers, kneeling, listening to drums or music, drinking wine, and holding hands, for example, are sensual experiences that enhance many rituals. Metaphoric materials often symbolize the four basic elements: fire, water, air, and earth. Their use may include lighting candles, pouring water, perfuming the air with burned herbs or incense, and arranging sand or eating/drinking the fruit of the earth. Hammerschlag and Silverman (1997) recommend "the talking circle," in which participants form a circle and speak in turn while holding a metaphoric object. Dress, another ritual ingredient, can be metaphoric (e.g, wearing bright, festive clothing to express joy and celebration) or convey a message (e.g., wearing a T-shirt with a personalized statement).
- A client may want to consider the role of ritual gift giving. Does the client want to inform participants that some type of gift is desired (e.g., a piece of advice, a comforting quote, or a flower)? Does the client want to present gifts to the participants?

Box 9-2 presents a case study application of the principles and practical considerations of creating a ceremonial ritual.

Box 9-2. One Client's Story: Healing Ritual

During a visit to a family practice clinic for an annual physical, Sharon Browne, age 21, confides to her nurse that a date rape experience she reported one year ago still makes her feel "dirty and contaminated." Because of her nurse's accepting and caring attitude, Sharon is able to describe a sense of deep anger about having been physically invaded and emotionally scarred against her will.

As her nurse actively listens, Sharon begins to realize that her response to victimization has a spiritual dimension. She recognizes

(continues)

Box 9-2. One Client's Story: Healing Ritual *(continued)*

that her anger is focused not only on her perpetrator but also on God ("for letting it happen"), others ("why should society let people get away with this?"), and herself ("I should have been less trusting").

Sharon yearns to feel that God does love her, that most people are worthy of trust, and that she can regain a sense of self-respect and worth. After expressing her spiritual distress, Sharon says, "I'm getting tired of carrying this anger around. It's like I want to wash away the dirtiness I feel and just get on with my life!"

When her nurse introduced the idea of creating a ritual to mark this transition, Sharon was enthusiastic. The nurse helped Sharon clarify the purpose of her ritual (i.e., to transition from feeling dirty and angry to clean and self-respectful) and then encouraged her to brainstorm about ways to symbolize this cleansing process. Although the nurse identified the different elements of a ritual, she made it clear that the ritual was for Sharon to plan.

Two weeks later, Sharon called to thank the nurse for her advice and encouragement—her spiritual caring. The nurse heard relief and buoyancy in Sharon's voice. Sharon reported what she had done to mark her transition from contaminated victim to clean survivor.

Sharon created a ritual for herself alone. First, she wrote down on paper as many things as she could identify that she wanted to "wash away." She bought a white negligee, candle, fragrant bath oil, and her favorite dessert. One evening, she filled her tub with warm water, added some fragrant oil, and lit the candle. She burned her list and got into the bath. While soaking, she imagined the water cleansing her emotionally and spiritually. As she stepped out of the bath, she symbolized her reentry into the world as a clean survivor by donning her new white negligee. Sharon then took time to write down a list of ways that her rape experience could make her a better person. She celebrated the transition by eating her dessert from a china plate.

Praying with Clients

Because praying with another person is a very intimate act, it should be approached carefully and respectfully. The nurse should introduce the intervention in a way that will be comfortable for both the client and the nurse. This introduction might include statements like: "Some people use prayer to cope with tough times like this. Would you feel comfortable if we prayed?" or "There is a growing amount of research that suggests that prayer is helpful, so I want you to know that I would be pleased to pray with or for you if you want. Just let me know."

To avoid praying with a client in an inappropriate manner, a brief assessment of the client's prayer habits is necessary. To whom does the client direct prayers? (Does the client address an Inner Light, Allah, or Jesus?) What type of prayer experience is comfortable for the present circumstances? (Does the client select a conversational prayer or a memorized ritual prayer that the nurse could repeat? Or does the client prefer a moment of shared silence?) Considering client personality may also indicate what types of prayer experience are most comforting. An extrovert may enjoy conversational prayer, for instance, and an introvert may prefer meditational prayer.

Another area to assess is what the client would like to pray for, information that may have been gathered during a prior conversation. A direct question like "For what would you like me to pray?" will likely bring a response that reveals the client's salient concerns.

When sharing a traditional, colloquial prayer with a client, remembering a few techniques may be helpful. Using the client's name and personalizing the prayer will make the client feel deeply cared for and heard. Speak for the client during the prayer. Give voice to his or her thoughts and feelings. At the conclusion, a client may want to reciprocate caring by voicing a prayer for the nurse. This gift should be received graciously; such gift giving is one of the few ways clients can reciprocate a nurse's care. It is not unusual for tears, hugs, or hand squeezes to follow prayer between two persons. The intimate experience of prayer can enhance the emotional bond between a nurse and a client.

Certain types of prayer may not be feasible. Excruciating pain or intense grief, for example, can often prevent a person from colloquial and meditative prayer. During such times, a ritual prayer may be most helpful. A short prayer or mantra that expresses the client's emotion and desire can be repeated, or a religious ritual prayer can be comforting. During times of intense crisis, it may be best to facilitate only those forms and approaches to prayer and meditation that are familiar and comfortable to the client.

While the intent of a nurse praying for a client may be compassionate, sensitivity to the client will help the nurse avoid creating discomfort for the client. There are times in life when clients may feel that their usual prayer practices are impossible or ineffective. Clients may experience spiritual doubts when they sense that they "can't pray anymore," question if they are "doing it right," wonder if it "does any good," or think "I'm not good enough to have my prayers answered" (Taylor et al., 1999). Suggesting to clients with such inner conflict that they pray, or pray more intensely or frequently, may contribute to spiritual distress. A client with such conflict about prayer may be best served by a spiritual care expert.

Prayer, especially traditional forms of prayer, can be used by professionals as a barrier to open communication with a client. Many chaplains, for example, recognize that clients sometimes request prayer to bring the visit to a speedy end. Sincere, caring people can also introduce prayer with a client when they feel uncomfortable with a client's sad circumstances or feel the need to physically or emotionally escape. Rather than use prayer to end an uncomfortable encounter, nurses should allow it to be a springboard for further discussion whenever it is appropriate.

Prayer should never function as a mechanism for propagandizing or enforcing a nurse's personal spiritual beliefs. Prayers like "God, please help Mrs. Smith to accept her illness," reflects a nurse's agenda rather than the client's if Mrs. Smith has indicated that she plans to "fight it!" A spoken prayer offered by a nurse should mirror—and give voice to—a client's innermost experience.

The experimental research involving intercessory prayer has raised ethical questions about the use of prayer as an intervention. Should someone pray for a client without his or her consent? Can a nurse in the privacy of his or her own mind maintain spiritual integrity and respect a personal belief by praying for a client even when the client has not requested prayer? Should a nurse pray for outcomes other than what the client desires? DeLashmutt and Silva (1998) concluded that nurses can ethically pray privately for a client, especially if they pray with an attitude of openness toward the will of God (or the Absolute). They base their argument on the fact that the nurse's intent is one of caring, that evidence is demonstrating the positive effects of prayer on health, and that most people would share the nurse's belief in prayer.

Box 9-3 provides samples of different types of prayer that a nurse can share with a client.

Box 9-3. Sample Prayers

Colloquial

"God, _____ is tired of being sick now. The pain in her stomach, the worrying about what is to come, the loneliness of being away from family, . . . [list concerns] . . . are beginning to overwhelm her. God, may wisdom and strength grow out of these worries and strains for _____ . Please God, may Your warm and comforting Presence be especially vivid for us now. We entrust _____ to You, the Creator and Sustainer of all of our lives, knowing that You will bring about what is ultimately good. Amen."

Petitionary

"God, please be with _____ in her sickness now. Ease the pain in her stomach, relieve her worry about the future, be close to her while she is separated from her family. We both want so much for her to be healed in whatever way You know is ultimately best. Please God, bless _____. Amen."

Meditational

A short phrase that helps a patient to commune with the divine can be selected (e.g., "Blessed be the Lord of my Salvation," "The Lord our God is One God," "God loves me") and the rest of Benson's steps to meditation can be followed.

A short passage of the patient's holy scripture can be read. The passage can be re-read slowly, allowing time for contemplation of subsections. The patient may be guided to consider certain questions while reflecting on the passage (e.g., How does this passage portray God in a way that is helpful to me now?). The patient may want to journal responses to the meditation.

The nurse may silently accompany a patient for a few minutes while each prays privately.

(continues)

Box 9-3. Sample Prayers (continued)

Ritual

Recitation or reading of a Psalm, such as the 23rd. Try inserting patient's name where pronouns are (e.g., "The Lord is Susan's Shepherd. She will not want. . . .").

"Lord Jesus Christ, Son of God, have mercy on me, a sinner." (This is an ancient, classic, Christian prayer that can easily be repeated during times of crisis.) The word *mercy* means (and may be substituted by) healing, wholeness, and love.

Facilitating Meditation

As with prayer, nurses can do several things for clients to facilitate meditation (e.g., protect client from unnecessary intrusions, schedule pain medications appropriately, bring a mandala or sacred music). Nurses can also provide instruction about meditation, such as Benson's steps for meditation practice. Helping clients to focus on their breathing and advising them about how to relate to extraneous thoughts are two specific ways nurses can assist clients with practicing meditation.

The focus on breathing is important to many approaches to meditation. After all, breathing—inspiration and expiration—are the essence of life and reflect and influence one's overall spirit. The ability to maintain deep, slow, rhythmic breathing improves with practice. Consideration of the client's respiratory condition, of course, is requisite before initiating such meditational techniques. To help a client establish this focused breathing, the nurse might say: "Slowly breathe in through your nose, counting 1 . . . 2 . . . 3 . . . hold that air inside a moment. Now breathe out through your mouth just as slowly, counting 1 . . . 2 . . . 3."

Although many approaches to meditation encourage a passive attitude toward distracting thoughts, Gill (1997) suggests that distractions can be stepping stones rather than stumbling blocks. Meditation is "the place where those normal, natural distractions can turn on the light and sound the gong to direct our attention to something within ourselves that we are afraid to face—but which God is inviting us to explore" (p. 13). For a client who complains that it is hard to concentrate while meditating because of distractions (e.g., feelings of anger or sexual images), the nurse can suggest that the distractions be reframed as indicators of inner exploration that is needed.

Using Imagery to Enhance Ritual

Imagery, the process of imagining that which is not being experienced directly, involves thinking that draws on the various senses (Achterberg, Dossey, & Kolkmeier, 1994). Although imagery is often equated with visualization in practice, imagining experiences visually is just one type of imagery. Imagery has also been described as a way of using the mind "to get in touch with the inner self" (Hoffart & Keene, 1998) and achieving "inner communication" (Tusek & Cwynar, 2000).

Techniques of imagery can also be useful for enhancing ritual. Before suggesting specific images to a client, the nurse conducts a brief assessment to gain useful information. People have different dominant senses and different life experiences that influence their imagination and how they interpret images. Helpful questions might include: What place would you find restful? When you try to imagine this place, what helps you most to sustain the image? The sounds? The smell? The picture of it?

The nurse may suggest spiritual images that bring comfort to a client. The image of God, an angel, Mary, or a favorite saint or other spiritual being can be incorporated in prayer. Imagining being in a sacred place may be meaningful for a client. Whatever the image, nurses can encourage clients to envision a wide range of physical aspects (e.g., what God is saying to them, how their angel's embrace feels, how the sacred space feels and sounds). Or clients may draw spiritual insight and comfort from imagining that they are the protagonist in a sacred story about healing (e.g., imagining that they are the hemorrhaging woman who touched Jesus's garment and became healed).

With imagery, it is essential that the client determine the metaphors and images. Not only will this image contain meaning specific to the client, but it will also avoid introducing negative side effects that could arise (e.g., imagining God as a comforting parent will likely be impossible for a survivor of parental abuse).

Imagery can be effectively combined with the focus on breathing during meditation. For example, while breathing in, the client might imagine absorbing forgiveness, love, or peace, and while breathing out imagine releasing shame, inferiority, or distress. Or a client might utter a ritual prayer that can be synchronized with the rhythm of breathing. The classic "Jesus prayer" many Christians recite might go like this: on inhalation, with a sense that Love is entering, "Lord, Jesus Christ, Son of God . . . ," on exhalation, with a sense that room is being made for healing, "have mercy on me, a sinner."

The preceding examples illustrate techniques that may alleviate spiritual distress. Spiritual images during prayers can also be very effective ways of coping with physical as well as emotional distress inherent in illness. Imagining the breath of God entering the body, going to a place of pain, and soothing it may be helpful. Or imagining Jesus as a companion during the lonely times of hospitalization may alleviate a Christian's loneliness.

Box 9-4 presents an interview with an expert nurse who regularly introduces imagery and meditation during her prayers with clients.

Box 9-4. One Nurse's Story: Using Meditative Prayer in Client Care

Katherine Brown-Saltzman, RN, MA, is a Palliative Care Nurse Specialist at the UCLA Medical Center. A large part of her practice involves attending to referrals she receives from health care professionals to request her healing methods that combine meditation, imagery, and prayer—or what Brown-Saltzman calls "meditative prayer."

How did you learn to pray in a meditative way?

The meditative prayer that I do has developed through the experiences of 25 years in nursing. It is my response to a gift I believe has been given to me by God. I also have a graduate degree that gave me expertise in intuition, imagery, and other techniques. So there are things that I do in my practice that are inappropriate for a novice to try.

Praying was a part of my family experience and my religious tradition. Earlier in my nursing career, I prayed with words. Responding to client requests, I would read Psalms and say ritual or intercessory prayers. But I reached a point when I felt that praying with words was not always effective. This seemed especially true when the client was from a tradition that differed from mine, was nonreligious, or an atheist. And then there were times when, for example, a client was suffering or in excruciating pain, that I was speechless. Didn't God already

Box 9-4. One Nurse's Story: Using Meditative Prayer in Client Care (continues)

know what was needed? Why do prayers need to be words, concrete thought?, I found myself asking. As these experiences with suffering clients shifted my thinking, I began to wonder what would happen if I just placed my hands on the client and thought about a blessing or whatever might be helpful for the client. My nursing practice already involved teaching clients relaxation techniques, imagery, and visualization. So I adapted these approaches to praying. Because spiritual care is so important to clients facing death, my work as a hospice and oncology nurse also inclined me in this direction.

How did you begin praying with clients?

I had always used touch with clients; I knew it to be very healing. So at times when I felt like there was nothing else to offer a client, I would hold his or her hand, or place my hand on the shoulder. Touch and praying have always been connected for me. After a personal experience of healing, I had the impression that I should touch clients on their sternum or chest while giving a blessing for them. I needed lots of courage, though, to do that! Even with my strong impression, it took me a while before I actually did it. Once I started doing this, I began to feel a vibration in my hands.

What do you "do" when you pray for a client? How do you pray?

First, I always ask about their spirituality. I usually say, "Can you tell me something about your spiritual beliefs?" Most clients indicate how religious they are, and some may share that they are not religious. I then explain the difference between spirituality and religion and what I offer, from generic relaxation strategies to meditative prayer, which I describe for them. I let them know that they can say "time out" for any reason.

If the client requests prayer, I place my hand on the chest (sternum), close my eyes, and remain open to that which guides me (in my framework, God). I may introduce an image. I may interact with the client about that image. I may move my hand(s) to wherever I sense healing needs to occur.

How do you care for a client who says he or she doesn't pray?

Meeting such a client is rare, but when I do, I review options that seem nonreligious (e.g., guided imagery). Sometimes, I have an over-

(continues)

Box 9-4. One Nurse's Story: Using Meditative Prayer in Client Care *(concluded)*

whelming sense that they do need prayer, and in my consciousness I go into that meditative state for them, even though I am fully engaged with them. The ethical dilemma for me is, "Do I pray for someone without their permission?" If during our initial interaction, a client makes a strong antireligious statement I don't offer prayer. Sometimes, however, the client will later request it. As one "nonbeliever" said to me, "I feel that there is something else, some energy, that you can give me."

What advice would you give to a nurse who wants to begin praying *with* clients?

Begin with a question to assess the client's spirituality. Start with clients with whom you are most comfortable (e.g., those who have a similar faith background), and then branch out as you feel called, comfortable. Talk with other health care professionals who pray with clients.

Describe a typical prayer experience with a client.

Oh, there are so many! There was a man with a mediastinal tumor who had left his religion and for whom illness represented a spiritual reawakening. When I offered meditational prayer, he was very responsive. I combined it with imagery, asking him to visualize a treasure chest and then to open it. When I placed my hand on his sternum, he said, "You've connected me to Someone Higher than myself."

With this man I had an image that he saw a book in his treasure chest. I sensed that I should tell him to read it, but my skepticism made me think, But what if he doesn't see a book in this treasure chest? Ignoring an insistent image, I said nothing. Later I asked him what he had found in his treasure chest. He said there had been a book. I asked if he'd opened it, and he said no. So I began to learn more about trusting my impressions.

The nurse's role is to teach clients about these techniques, and possibly to coach or guide them as they begin. Approaches presented in this chapter are relatively simple and unlikely to elicit negative side effects. As with any spiritual care intervention, however, the nurse needs to be aware of the possibility that serious spiritual or emotional issues may be brought to a conscious level and will then require referral to an expert.

KEY POINTS

- Rituals involve repetition, special or stylized behavior, order, an evocative presentation, and a collective dimension. Rituals support people spiritually by enabling them to relate, change, heal, believe, and celebrate.
- Different types of prayer include: meditational, conversational, petitionary, and ritual. Prayer is also categorized by its intent (e.g., expression of gratitude, lament, or request).
- Although research indicating positive health benefits from intercessory prayer is limited, there is ample evidence that clients often use prayer as a coping strategy.
- Research suggests that clients may want their health care professionals to pray with them and that many nurses do pray privately for clients.
- Effective use of ritual to nurture client spiritual health is characterized by:
  - Adequate assessment to determine client perception of need and appropriateness of nurse participation in planning the ritual.
  - Keeping rituals simple and associating them with common daily occurrences.
  - Attending to several areas when planning a ritual: purpose, outside pressures, preparation, people, place, "sacraments," participation, and gifts.
- Suggestions for practicing prayer with clients include creating personalized conversational prayers that reflect current concerns and matching the type of prayer experience with the client's personality, preference, and current circumstance.

- Praying with clients is an effective intervention when the nurse is able to:

  ○ Recognize that prayer experiences need to be flexible, matched with the client's needs.

  ○ Use prayer as a springboard for discussion, rather than as a mechanism for ending an uncomfortable conversation.

  ○ Praying with an open-ended, loving, "Thy will be done" attitude, rather than invoking magic.

  ○ Resist using prayer as a vehicle for preaching or pushing a personal agenda.

- Meditation is a ritual that may or may not recognize the presence of a divine entity. Benson (1997) concluded that maintaining a passive, alert focus on a meaningful thought was essential to eliciting a relaxed state during meditation.

- Imagery, the process of imagining that which is not being directly experienced, aids meditation and prayer.

LOOK WITHIN TO LEARN

1. What rituals do you practice daily, weekly, yearly, or less frequently? In what ways do these rituals sustain you spiritually?

2. How do you respond to rituals that no longer hold meaning for you? Do you avoid them, revise them, or continue "to go through the motions"?

3. What does prayer mean to you? Does the way you pray nurture you spiritually? What other types of prayer experience might be helpful to you?

4. What meditation and imagery techniques might you find helpful?

5. How have difficult life experiences shaped the way you participate in rituals, including prayer? When you were "really down" or facing a crisis, what type of ritual or prayer was (or would have been) helpful?

REFERENCES

Bold print indicates those that are most recommended.

Achterberg, J., Dossey, B., & Kolkmeier, L. (1994). Rituals of healing: Using imagery for health and wellness. New York: Bantam Books.

Ai, A. L., Dunkle, R. E., Peterson, C., & Bolling, S. F. (1998). The role of private prayer in psychological recovery among midlife and aged patients following cardiac surgery. *Gerontologist, 38*(5), 591–601.

Anselmo, J., & Kolkmeier, L. G. (2000). Relaxation: The first step to restore, renew, and self-heal. In B. M. Dossey, L. Keegan, & C. E. Guzzetta (Eds.), *Holistic Nursing: A handbook for practice* (3rd ed., pp. 497–535). Gaithersburg, MD: Aspen.

Armstrong, R. D. (1998, August/September). First the body, then the mind: Effective rituals spring from the depths. *The Park Ridge Center Bulletin*, 5.

Ashby, L. S., & Lenhart, R. S. (1994). Prayer as a coping strategy for chronic pain patients. *Rehabilitation Psychology, 39*, 205–209.

Astin, J. A., Harkness, E., & Ernst, E. (2000). The efficacy of "distant healing": A systematic review of randomized trials. *Annals of Internal Medicine, 132*, 903–910.

Bearon, L. B., & Koenig, H. G. (1990). Religious cognitions and use of prayer in health and illness. *Gerontologist, 30*(2), 249–253.

Benson, H. (1997). *Timeless healing: The power and biology of belief.* New York: Scribners.

Boisset, M., & Fitzcharles, M. (1994). Alternative medicine use by rheumatology patients in a universal health care setting. *Journal of Rheumatology, 21*, 148–152.

Byrd, R. C. (1988). Positive therapeutic effects of intercessory prayer in a coronary care unit population. *Southern Medical Journal, 81*(7), 826–829.

Carson, V. B. (1993). Prayer, meditation, exercise, and special diets: Behaviors of the hardy person with HIV/AIDS. *Journal of the Association of Nurses in AIDS Care, 4*(3), 18–28.

Conversations: Larry Dossey, MD: Healing and the nonlocal mind: Interview by Bonnie Horrigan (1999). *Alternative Therapies in Health and Medicine, 5*(6), 85–93.

DeLashmutt, M., & Silva, M. C. (1998). Ethical issues: The ethics of long-distance intercessory prayer. *Nursing Connections, 11*(4): 37–40.

Dossey, L. (1993). *Healing words: The power of prayer and the practice of medicine.* San Francisco: HarperSanFrancisco.

Eisenberg, D. M., Kessler, R. C., Foster, C., Norlock, F. E., Calkins, D. R., & Delbanco, T. L. (1993). Unconventional medicine in the United States: Prevalence, costs, and patterns of use. *New England Journal of Medicine, 328*, 246–252.

Froggatt, K. (1997). Signposts on the journey: The place of ritual in spiritual care. *International Journal of Palliative Nursing, 3*(1), 42–46.

Gallup, G. H., Jr. (1996). *Religion in America*. Princeton, NJ: Princeton Religion Research Center.

Gill, S. D. (1987). Prayer. In M. Eliade (Ed.), *The encyclopedia of religion*. (pp. 489–492). New York: Macmillan.

Gill, J. (1997). Distraction in prayer: Stumbling blocks or stepping stones? *Presence: The Journal of Spiritual Directors International, 3*(1), 6–18.

Hammerschlag, C. A., & Silverman, H. D. (1997). Healing ceremonies: Creating personal rituals for spiritual, emotional, physical, and mental healing. New York: Perigee.

Harris, W. S., Gowda, M., Kolb, J. W., Strychacz, C. P., Vacek, J. L., Jones, P. G., et al. (1999). A randomized, controlled trial of the effects of remote, intercessory prayer on outcomes in patients admitted to the coronary care unit. *Archives of Internal Medicine, 159*, 2273–2278.

Hoffart, M. B., & Keene, E. P. (1998). Body–mind–spirit: The benefits of visualization. *American Journal of Nursing, 98*(12), 44–47.

Imber-Black, E., & Roberts, J. (1993). *Rituals for our times: Celebrating, healing, and changing our lives and our relationships.* New York: HarperPerennial.

King, D. E., & Bushwick, B. (1994). Beliefs and attitudes of hospital inpatients about faith healing and prayer. *Journal of Family Practice, 39,* 349–352.

King, M. O., Pettigrew, A., & Reed, F. C. (2000). Complementary, alternative, integrative: Have nurses kept pace with their clients? *Dermatology Nursing, 12*(1), 41–44, 47–50.

Levin, J. S. (1996). How prayer heals: A theoretical model. *Alternative Therapies in Health and Medicine, 2*(1), 66–73.

Levin, J. S., Lyons, J. S., & Larson, D. B. (1993). Prayer and health during pregnancy: Findings from the Galveston low birthweight survey. *Southern Medical Journal, 86*(9), 1022–1027.

May, G. G. (1982). *Care of mind: Care of spirit: Psychiatric dimensions of spiritual direction.* San Francisco: Harper & Row.

McRoberts, J. M., Sato, A., & Southwick, W. E. (2000). Spiritual care: A study on the views and practices of psychiatric nurses. *Research for Nursing Practice.* Available on-line at http://www.graduateresearch.com/mcroberts.htm.

Meisenhelder, J. B., & Chandler, E. N. (2000). Prayer and health outcomes in church members. *Alternatives Therapies in Health and Medicine, 6*(4), 56–60.

Ohaeri, J., Shokunbi, W., Akinlade, K., & Dare, L. (1995). The psychosocial problems of sickle cell disease sufferers and their methods of coping. *Social Science and Medicine, 40,* 955–960.

O'Laoire, S. (1997). An experimental study of the effects of distant, intercessory prayer on self-esteem, anxiety, and depression. *Alternative Therapies in Health and Medicine, 3*(6), 38–42, 44–53.

Oyama, O., & Koenig, H. G. (1998). Religious beliefs and practices in family medicine. *Archives of Family Medicine, 7,* 431–435.

Peteet, J. R., Stomper, P. C., Ross, D. M., Cotton, V., Turesdell, P., & Moczynski, W. (1992). Emotional support for patients with cancer who are undergoing CT: Semistructured interviews of patients at a cancer institute. *Radiology, 182*(1), 99–102.

Poloma, M. M., & Gallup, G. H., Jr. (1991). *Varieties of prayer: A survey report.* Philadelphia: Trinity Press.

Richards, D. G. (1991). The phenomenology and psychological correlates of verbal prayer. *Journal of Psychology and Theology, 19,* 354–363.

Roberts, L., Ahmed, I., Hall, S., & Sargent, C. (2000). Intercessory prayer for the alleviation of ill health. *The Cochrane Library (Oxford),* issue 1. (Update software, online or CD-ROM).

Rozanski, J. K. (1997). *Prayer and critical care nursing.* Unpublished master's thesis. Miami: Florida International University.

Saudia, T. L., Kinney, M. R., Brown, K. C., & Young-Ward, L. (1991). Health locus of control and helpfulness of prayer. *Heart & Lung, 20*(1), 60–65.

Stolley, J. M., Buckwalter, K. C., & Koenig, H. G. (1999). Prayer and religious coping for caregivers of persons with Alzheimer's disease and related disorders. *American Journal of Alzheimer's Disease, 14*(3), 181–191.

Sutton, T. D., & Murphy, S. P. (1989). Stressors and patterns of coping in renal transplant patients. *Nursing Research, 38*(1), 46–49.

Targ, E. (1997). Evaluating distant healing: A research review. *Alternative Therapies in Health & Medicine, 3*(6), 74–78.

Taylor, A. G., Lin, Y., Snyder, A., & Eggleston, K. (1998). ED staff members' personal use of complementary therapies and their recommendations to ED patients. A southeastern US regional survey. *Journal of Emergency Nursing, 24*(pp. 495–499).

Taylor, E. J., Amenta, M., & Highfield, M. F. (1995). Spiritual care practices of oncology nurses. *Oncology Nursing Forum, 22*(1), 31–39.

Taylor, E. J., Outlaw, F. H., Bernardo, T. R., & Roy, A. (1999). Spiritual conflicts associated with praying about cancer. *Psycho-Oncology, 8,* 386–394.

Tusek, D. L., & Cwynar, R. E. (2000). Strategies for implementing a guided imagery program to enhance patient experience. *AACN Clinical Issues: Advanced Practice in Acute & Critical Care, 11*(1), 68–76.

Ulanov, A., & Ulanov, B. (1982). *Primary speech: A psychology of prayer.* Atlanta, GA: John Knox Press.

Webster, D. C., & Brennan, T. (1995). Self-care strategies used for acute attack of interstitial cystitis. *Urologic Nursing, 15*(3), 86–93.

Wierzbicka, A. (1994). What is prayer? In search of a definition. In L. B. Brown (Ed.). *The human side of prayer.* (Chapter 2, pp. 25–46). Birmingham, AL: Religious Education Press.

10

Facilitating
Religious Practices

Most Americans are religious. Although only 69 percent of adults claim membership in a religious body, 92 percent state a religious preference. Religion is valued by Americans: 58 percent acknowledge that religion is very important, and 30 percent indicate that it is the most important aspect of their lives (Gallup, 1996).

Religion, which offers codified beliefs supported by a social organization, is used by people to express their spirituality. Religion also provides a structured means for discovering and developing one's spirituality and represents a fundamental aspect of the lives of many clients. It is important for the nurse to become familiar with religious beliefs and practices. Religious beliefs influence how a client interprets life experiences, illness, and death, as well as client attitudes and behaviors regarding personal health. Health challenges and medical treatments in turn may affect a client's ability to practice religion.

This chapter summarizes relevant research, presents an overview of characteristics of selected religions, and explores how the nurse facilitates client religious practices.

HEALTH BENEFITS OF RELIGIOUS PRACTICE

Most of the hundreds of studies that explore the connection between religiosity and physical and mental health have demonstrated a positive relationship. In response to the question posed by his book title, "Is religion good for your health?" Koenig (1997) asserts that it is. Koenig reviews research that documents positive relationships between religiosity and physical and mental well-being for persons of all ages. While Jarvis and Northcott (1987) concluded, after reviewing research on the influence of religiosity on morbidity and mortality, that it is impossible to make grand statements affirming a definite relationship between these factors, they did recognize that "it is becoming evident that religion has a powerful effect on the way many people live, on the quality of their life, and on the length of time they live to experience that quality" (p. 822).

Levin (1994; Levin & Schiller, 1987) also presented a thorough analysis of hundreds of studies of religion and health and concluded that an association exists between religion and health. Levin suggested that the answer to the question of whether the association is valid (i.e., not due to chance) is "probably" and whether religion can cause healthful outcomes is "maybe."

Matthews and colleagues (1998) reached similar conclusions: Religious commitment or involvement appears to play a role in illness prevention, recovery from illness, and coping with an illness. They identified clusters of research reports supporting a link between religious commitment and decreased prevalence of depression, substance abuse, and physical illness such as hypertension. Religious commitment may also increase longevity. These authors conclude that physicians should inquire about and, if appropriate, encourage a client's religiosity.

Meta-analyses more often than not reveal a positive relationship between mental health and religiosity. Koenig (1997), for example, generalized that those who are more religious are less anxious and depressed, deal better with adversity, and are less likely to abuse alcohol. Gartner, Larson, and Allen (1991) identified several additional mental health factors that are positively related to religious commitment, including increased marital satisfaction and a lower incidence of divorce, suicide, drug use, and delinquency. Larson and colleagues (1992) observed that studies investigating the ceremonial and social dimensions of spirituality, prayer, and relationship with God consistently reported beneficial associations with mental health.

Pargament's (1997) review of research substantiates that persons facing challenging circumstances often benefit from religious coping strategies. Pargament summarized dozens of research studies with findings about religious coping. Hupcey's (2000) qualitative study of intensive care unit patients, for example, illustrates how religious beliefs can be an essential source of comfort that some clients will describe as "what has gotten me through."

Levin (1994) hypothesized several mechanisms that individually or in combination may explain the health benefits derived from religiosity. These include:

- **Behavior:** Many religions advocate behaviors and lifestyles known to promote health (e.g., vegetarianism, abstinence from smoking, alcohol, drugs, and extramarital sex).
- **Psychosocial effects:** Active participation in a religious group brings social support, a sense of belonging, and fellowship. Social support has been well established as a factor linked with health.
- **Psychodynamics of belief systems:** Religious belief may bring a person a sense of peacefulness, self-confidence, purpose—positive feelings that in turn support physiologic well-being. Religious beliefs may also inspire negative feelings, like guilt, that can harm health.

- **Psychodynamics of faith:** The effects of placing faith in a God or religion, trusting biblical promises, and so forth, may contribute to health.
- **Psychodynamics of religious rites:** Participating in religious worship may reduce anxiety and produce emotional arousal or a sense of being loved within a community, which can have a placebo-like effect on health.
- **Superempirical force:** Accessing a force or energy (e.g., chi, prana, life force, God's spirit) may explain the connection between religiosity and health.

RELIGIOUS CHALLENGES TO HEALTH CARE

Although religion characteristically promotes health and supports coping, it is possible that some religious beliefs may interfere with traditional approaches to providing health care. In some situations, certain religious beliefs may even be deleterious to health. Nurses have recognized the potential for harmful effects of specific religious beliefs on client responses to illness (Taylor, Highfield, & Amenta, 1994). A survey of oncology nurses (n = 146) that asked how client beliefs can be a hindrance to health indicated two categories: (1) religious beliefs that restrict the use of medical interventions (e.g., Jehovah's Witnesses who disapprove of administration of blood products) and (2) religious beliefs that bring psychological harm (e.g., viewing disease as a result of sin and evidence of God's wrath toward a client). A client who refuses pain medication and states "My pain is God's will" illustrates this phenomenon (Kumasaka, 1996) as do families who insist on medical intervention for aggressive end-of-life care "so that God can work a miracle" (Connors & Smith, 1996).

While forcefully arguing the merits of religion in the coping process, Pargament (1997) suggested that certain religious beliefs may hinder healthful responses to negative life events when they prevent a client from:

- Being able to draw on a variety of coping responses to a situation
- Having flexibility to interpret religious practices and beliefs
- Behaving in a manner that is consistent with personally held beliefs
- Experiencing a sense of secure attachment to God

Hufford's (1993) study of popular theologies of healing among Christians contrasts potentially helpful and harmful beliefs. Hufford identified two categories of thinking, which he labeled: "You will be healed," and "You may be healed." The position that "You may be healed" accepts that God's will is good, but mysterious, and that suffering is a result of sin's existing in the world. Clients with this stance will accept medical care as a way in which God can heal; if physical cure does not occur, they accept that whatever happens is spiritually best. The other position contends that God, who wills all to be healthy, will heal. Such a position leads to an attitude that health care is superfluous and seeking it demonstrates lack of faith; it also correlates with the belief that if healing does not occur, it is because one is still in a state of sin or not praying correctly. It is this latter position that typically creates dilemmas for nurses.

REVIEW OF SELECTED RELIGIOUS BELIEFS AND PRACTICES

Nursing care is more effective when it is informed by at least some knowledge of various religious traditions that influence client attitudes toward health and health care. A variety of religious traditions flourish in North America. Box 10-1 presents membership statistics.

Box 10-1. North American Religions	
Religion	**Membership**
Baptist (including Southern, General, Progressive, Conservative, and other Baptist denominations)	19,665,000
Buddhism	401,000
Churches of Christ (including Disciples of Christ and United Church of Christ)	5,685,000
Eastern Orthodox (e.g., Coptic, Serbian, and Greek Orthodox, Armenian Apostolic)	5,270,000
Episcopal	2,537,000
Hinduism	227,000
Islam (Muslim)	527,000
Jehovah's Witnesses	976,000
Judaism	3,137,000

Box 10-1. North American Religions *(continued)*	
Latter Day Saints (Mormons, including Reorganized LDS)	4,978,000
Lutheran (including Missouri, Wisconsin synods, and Evangelical)	8,195,000
Mennonite, Church of the Brethren, and Amish	496,000
Methodist & Wesleyan	8,613,000
Methodist Episcopal	5,471,000
Pentecostal and Holiness (including Assemblies of God, Free Methodist, Church of the Nazarene, various Churches of God, Salvation Army)	8,819,000
Presbyterian and Reformed denominations	4,504,000
Roman Catholic	61,208,000
Seventh-day Adventist	809,000
Unitarian Universalist	502,000
Other fundamental or evangelical Christian denominations (e.g., Foursquare, Gospel Fellowships, Evangelical Free Church)	1,008,000

Note: Some groups may be excluded if they did not supply information or have a small membership.

Source: U.S. Census Bureau. (1998). Statistical abstract of the United States (Table no. 89). Available online: http://www.census.gov.

The following provides an overview of key religions. For further information, the reader can consult an encyclopedia of religion or two books that discuss health and medicine from the perspective of various world religious traditions (i.e., Numbers & Amundsen, 1986; Sullivan, 1989).

Buddhism

Founded in the sixth century before the common era (B.C.E.) in India by Siddhartha Gautama, who became known as Buddha, Buddhism spread throughout Asia over the next several centuries. Today, many Americans have adopted Buddhist teaching. Clients who practice Buddhism, however, are more likely to be from a Chinese, Korean, Japanese, or southeastern Asian culture.

Beliefs

Although variations exist among many subdivisions of Buddhism, some teachings of Buddha are central to all. Buddhist commitment is summed in the "three jewels": worship of Buddha; obedience to laws and teachings ("dharma," which are passed orally and in numerous, lengthy tomes); and support for communities of monks. Buddha presented the prescription for spiritual health in his "Four Noble Truths": (1) Everything in the world is suffering and sorrow; (2) suffering results from the desire for attachment, satisfaction, and permanence even though everything about life and the self is transient; (3) when desire is eliminated, suffering ends and one reaches Nirvana; and (4) the way to end desire is to follow the "Eightfold Path." Buddhists believe that this path helps those who follow it to become enlightened and move closer to Nirvana. This path means striving to understand suffering, renounce all attachments, express oneself lovingly, behave correctly, avoid hurting others, work toward spiritual growth, develop the ability to reflect on personal experience, and establish perfect intellectual concentration.

Buddists believe in the theory of "karma," that for every action there is a consequence, and the consequence will occur either in this or a future life. Some Buddhist clients believe that their health problems are attributable to poor choices made during a previous life that created negative karma. Because Buddhists believe in reincarnation, they feel it is acceptable to miss someone who dies but inappropriate to mourn, because death actually allows rebirth.

Practices

Because diverse cultures influence its application to life, Buddhist practices vary widely. Most Buddhists are not ascetic monks or nuns seeking Nirvana, but lay people who strive toward moral conduct in this life and improved circumstances in the next life. Regular meditation, chanting, preparing an altar graced by a Buddha, making pilgrimages to sacred places, attending temple for instruction, vegetarianism, and avoiding alcohol, tobacco, and nonmedicinal drugs are practices reflective of Buddhist tradition that may be followed by a Buddhist client.

Originally a nontheistic philosophy, Buddhism has been influenced by other religio-cultural systems. Thus, some Buddhists may pray in a petitionary way to a god. Objects used during prayer or meditation may include mandalas, bells or gongs, and prayer beads. Although tomes of sacred writings and analyses of these writings reflect Buddhist tradition, there is no "Buddhist Bible."

Christianity

Christianity originated as a Jewish sect whose members believed that Jesus was the promised messiah. Not until after Jesus died on a cross, was witnessed to have been resurrected and ascended to Heaven, and his following began to grow was the title *Christ* commonly used for Jesus and *Christians* for his followers. Christianity, found in many places around the world, is the pervading religion of Europe, Australia, and North and South America.

Beliefs

Most Christians believe in three dimensions of God, or a Trinity, known traditionally as Father, Holy Spirit, and Jesus. Jesus, considered by Christians to be the personification of God, is perceived to have been simultaneously divine and human in nature during his life on earth. Because of his death and resurrection (30 or 33 C.E.), those who believe in him feel that they will have the opportunity for salvation (i.e., reconciliation with God). While Christians hold different views on what occurs after death, they generally accept that there is an afterlife and that God's final judgment determines an individual's ultimate future (e.g., heaven or hell).

Practices

Christians regard Old and New Testaments of the Bible as sacred, inspired scripture. Two characteristic rituals are communion (or Eucharist, the ingestion of bread and wine as symbols of Jesus's body and blood) and baptism (an immersion or application of water to signify cleansing from sin and passage into Christianity). As with other major faith traditions, Christianity has been shaped by diverse cultures. It has grown to encompass numerous denominations, and nurses will frequently encounter clients from these denominations.

Hinduism

Hinduism emerged as a religion among the people of India around 1500 B.C.E. Hindu clients whom nurses encounter generally will have emigrated from India or be descendants of those who have. Enmeshed with Indian culture, Hinduism is as varied in its interpretations as are the Indian people.

Beliefs

Hindus believe Brahman is an omniscient, omnipresent, and omnipotent God, whose roles are represented in the trinity of Brahma (God as creator), Vishnu (God as preserver), and Shiva (God as destroyer). Both Vishnu and Shiva are portrayed and worshipped in thousands of guises, making Hinduism a polytheistic religion. Hindus derive guidance from over 200 holy books (including the Vedas and Upanishads). The most revered is the Bhagavad Gita, a book of poetry describing a warrior's crisis of conscience, which identifies paths for the Hindu to find union with God. These ways of life include seeking practical and spiritual knowledge, acting with detachment toward the fruits of one's labor and offering it to God, and devotion to God.

Hindus believe in reincarnation, that the soul persists even though the body changes, dies, and is reborn. This soul may return in different forms, including that of an animal, depending on the law of karma. The cycle of reincarnation ends when one reaches the spiritual goal of abandoning all desires and attachments, a state of being characterized as union with God (Brahman).

Practices

The Hindu religious calendar includes numerous festivals, fasts, and holidays. Along with these holy days, some Hindus may observe on specific days of each week worship for certain gods. For reasons of compassion, many Hindus are vegetarians. Most Hindu families have a chosen god, called an "Ishta Deva," who protects and blesses their home. Many maintain a shrine in the home with items such as a picture of Shiva or other god, oil lamp, incense, bell, scripture, prayer beads, photograph of a guru, and gifts of fruit and flowers for the god. Yoga, the use of mantras, mandalas and yantras (three-dimensional geometric objects that offer a focus for worship), and pilgrimages to holy cities or rivers are other practices Hindus exercise to find union with God.

Islam

Islam was founded early in the seventh century in what is now Saudi Arabia by Muhammad after he received a vision from God. Because missionary efforts are part of the Moslem expression of faith, Islam is found around the world. Moslem clients often will be native to Asia, Africa, the Middle East, Europe, or North America.

Beliefs

Islam's central tenet is expressed in the often cited "There is no God but God, and Muhammad is his messenger." That is, there is only one God (in Arabic, "Allah"), and this God is a personal god that humans can approach directly in prayer. Fundamental Islamic doctrine also includes belief in angels as God's messengers, in God as having predetermined life for people, and in a resurrection of the dead at the end of time with a final judgment by God determining whether individuals enter heaven or hell. Sharia, or the directive for how Moslems should live, declares five goals for believers: to protect life, mind, religion, family, and property. A health care decision would thus be determined ultimately by the goal of protecting life. Islamic sacred writings include the visions and teachings of Muhammad as found in the Koran and the living commentary based on the Koran found in the Hadith.

Practices

The most fundamental Islamic religious practices are those identified in the "Five Pillars of Faith." The first pillar is the confession of faith. The second pillar calls the believer to pray at dawn, noon, afternoon, sunset, and night while facing the city of Mecca (Saudi Arabia). These prayers ideally are said in mosques, where women pray separately from men. The prayers are preceded by ritual ablutions (i.e., washing hands, face, and feet, and performing certain movements). The third pillar mandates that believers fast daily from dawn to sunset during the month of Ramadan (determined by the lunar calendar). Travelers, pregnant or ill persons, and the elderly are exempted from this fast, which includes abstinence from food, water, and sex. The fourth pillar requires Moslems to give "alms" or charity (e.g., help the sick). The fifth pillar stipulates that, if possible, a pilgrimage to Mecca should be made at least once during one's lifetime.

The Moslem's holy day is Friday. Believers generally attend a worship service that begins at noon and is led by an imam, the local spiritual leader. When a client wishes to pray in traditional Moslem style, desired objects can include a prayer mat, hat, beads, and compass (to determine the location of Mecca).

Judaism

Judaism is the religion of Jewish people (and converts). Although not all Jews practice Judaism, those who do may observe the religion with different degrees of orthodoxy (i.e., from Ultra Orthodox to Modern Orthodox, Conservative, Reconstructionist, Reformed, and Ultra Reformed). Although Judaism's date of origin is uncertain, significant early events include the call of Abraham (who can be credited with founding Christianity and Islam, as well as Judaism), God giving the Jews the Ten Commandments at Sinai and signifying them as a chosen people, an exile of the Jews that began in 586 B.C.E., and the destruction of the Temple in Jerusalem in 70 C.E. (commemorated on Tishah B'Ab). Today, practicing Jews live primarily in Israel, Europe, and the United States (especially in large Eastern cities and Los Angeles).

Beliefs

The beliefs of Judaism may be summarized in the credos: "Hear O Israel, The Lord is our God, The Lord is one" and "Love God . . . with all your heart and with all your soul" (Deuteronomy 6:5–9). Judaism accepts that God is the creator and sustainer of the universe. God created people, provided them with guidance and free will to choose between good and evil, and gives redemption, salvation, and an ultimate justice after life. Because YHWH, or Yahweh, is the most sacred of terms used to refer to God, no Jew will ever pronounce it; instead, terms like Adonai, Lord, or "the Holy One, blessed be He" are used.

Although Judaism recognizes an afterlife, the nature of this afterlife remains undefined. Judaism also teaches that there will be a messiah; however, whether this will be a divinely sent messenger or a movement that ushers peace into the world is debated. Beliefs are drawn from the Jewish Bible and tradition. The Jewish Bible (what Christians refer to as the Old Testament) is composed of the Law (or Torah), Prophets, and Writings. Tradition is largely embodied in the volumes of the Talmud, the collected oral law and rabbinic commentaries.

Practices

Judaic practices reflect 613 mitzvot, or commands of God, found in the Torah. The mitzvah provide direction for how to relate to God (e.g., when and how to worship) and to others (e.g., prescriptives for ethical behavior, being charitable to the poor). Perhaps the most distinctive mitzvot are the command to rest and worship on Shabbat and to "keep kosher" (i.e., to prepare and eat food according to the dietary laws). Several religious holidays occur throughout the year, when observant Jews will likely attend synagogue and utilize or make certain symbolic objects or foods.

Native American Religiosity

Although there is a resurgent interest in Native American religion, the religious oppression (1887–1934) of Native Americans served to distance them from their traditional practices (Deloria, 1994). Prior to the invasion of Westerners, Native Americans lived in tribes, of which there were more than 300, and each tribe developed a unique form of religion. Because many tribes have been eradicated or merged and many Native Americans have assimilated to Western religions, much of this religious practice has been lost. Today, some forms of religion cross tribal lines (e.g., the Native American Church).

Beliefs

Native American life—culture, politics, history, society—is enmeshed with religion. The purpose of various forms of Native American religion is to understand how to relate as a community of people (i.e., a tribe) with other living things. Native Americans seek to develop the self-discipline necessary to behave harmoniously with other creatures, which include animals, plants, and sometimes inanimate objects of the earth. They recognize their dependence on the natural world, and base their actions and ethics on a sense of moral responsibility toward this world. Death is viewed as a passage from one form of experience to another, a change in worlds. In death, a person's body becomes the soil that sustains life for other creatures. Religion, rather than an individualistic relationship with a higher power, is a covenant between a tribe and a particular god. Native American religions recognize various good and evil spiritual entities (e.g., ghosts, gods, spirits of ancestors) within nature. They also acknowledge a higher God, sometimes called the Great Spirit, or Wakan Tanka. Disease and injury are explained by a weakened relationship with the supernatural world.

Practices

Because harmony with the natural world forms the core of Native American religions, rituals and ceremonies are dependent on sacred spaces such as rivers, mountains, and places linked with a significant event for the tribe or where Native Americans have long gone to commune with higher spiritual powers. Sacred places and ceremonial rituals are considered private and are usually kept secret from those outside the tribe. Common components of sacred ceremonies include singing or chanting occasion-specific songs, drumming, dancing, and "other peoples" (i.e., plants, animals). Healing ceremonies may incorporate the use of roots, herbs, or other plants gathered from a sacred place. Today, in addition to Native American political leaders elected to serve, spiritual leaders, medicine men, and shamans also provide assistance (e.g., foretelling and general advice, healing) for tribal members.

SYNCRETISTIC RELIGIONS

Over the past millennia, unique religions have arisen from the merging of other religious and cultural belief systems (i.e., syncretism). Sikhism, for example, is a merging of Hindu and Islamic traditions. The Baha'i Faith reflects Islamic belief and nineteenth-century culture. Black Muslims incorporate Islam and twentieth-century African American ideology in the religion of the Nation of Islam. Christian Science incorporates ancient Hindu and Western Christian thinking. Theosophy recognizes ancient Gnostic theology and Eastern concepts like karma and reincarnation. The Unification Church espouses Christianity mixed with Taoist philosophy. This continual creation of new religions demonstrates the timeless, innate, global phenomenon of religion as a spiritual search (Allan, 1994).

The term *New Age* has been used to designate another syncretistic religious movement, prevalent in American society during the 1980s and 1990s. New Age thinking encompasses ancient astrological ideas, Eastern philosophies and practices, and Christianity. Allan (1994) summarized the New Age message as "We are more than we imagine. If only we can understand our divinity, and our oneness with all creation, we can bring peace to ourselves and contribute to the evolution of our planet" (p. 405). This New Age worldview is supported by a belief that everything in the universe is unified, that in reality everything is interrelated, synergistic. It is also based on the notion of pantheism, that everything is God and God is in everything. Thus, the distinction between God and human is blurred. Accepting that the Divine is within, New Age believers seek to reconnect to that perfect love, wisdom, and intelligence. Spiritual practices used by New Age believers include Eastern forms of meditation, channeling (i.e., mentally making energy transform to a more dense frequency in order to find greater personal clarity and direction), and wearing crystals and gemstones (thought to magnify energy) (Doyne, 1990).

SPIRITUALITY OF THE NONRELIGIOUS

Some clients will describe themselves as "not religious." They may be atheists, individuals who are without a belief in a God or gods. They may be agnostics, doubting the existence of God. Many atheists and agnostics are considered to be secular humanists who emphasize the use of the scientific method and critical thinking to better human life and reject claims of any paranormal experiences. For secular humanists, the existence of God cannot be logically proven. Although their conduct is not guided by specific religious principles, they value developing a moral code for themselves. The Golden Rule, for example, may guide them to determine what is right and wrong.

Nonreligious clients may include those who have never explored religion or have come from a religious background but have withdrawn from or even become antagonistic toward religion. Some people have felt betrayed by a religious person, cleric, or God, often leaving them with a deep-seated bitterness or the tendency to generalize that all religion is bad. A person may have parents or grandparents who were religious but for some reason withdrew from religiosity and did not transmit it to the next generation. Many teens and young adults, as a natural part of spiritual development (see Chapter 1), reevaluate the religion of their parents, and in the process of developing spiritually, find that the religiosity of their childhood no longer holds meaning for them. While some may seek a meaningful religiosity, others choose to avoid or abandon religion.

Nonreligious clients, like all people, have a spiritual dimension, reflected in universal striving for meaningfulness and purpose; love and belonging; harmony with self, nature, and others; and peace. Thus, a nonreligious client's need for spiritual care is no different from that of a religious person (Burnard, 1988). An agnostic 19-year-old man receiving cancer treatments, for example, may find spiritual healing by practicing meditation to quiet himself and "get in touch with what he needs to be and do." An atheist client receiving hospice care may choose to cope with spiritual despair about dying by sleeping as much as possible.

Because theistic religio-cultural systems exert marked sociocultural influence, nonreligious clients may not feel comfortable talking openly about personal beliefs. Approaching a nonreligious client requires sensitivity, especially if the nurse is unfamiliar with the nonreligious experience. Although it may be appropriate for the nurse to change the subject when a nonreligious client reacts with anger when the topic of spirituality is raised, the nurse should view an angry response as a clue rather than a reason to flee. An argumentative or defensive response from the nurse is inappropriate, of course.

COMMON RELIGIOUS PRACTICES

Facilitating a client's wish to observe religious practices requires some degree of prior assessment. Clients observe religious practices based on their knowledge and interpretation of, as well as their commitment to, their religion. Interpretations can range from conservative and orthodox to liberal and unorthodox. Commitment to religious practices can range from strong to weak. A client's religious practice is influenced by a number of factors including the religiosity of family of origin, cultural influences, personality, the degree of diversity encouraged by the religion, and life experiences. Thus, to some degree, each client practices his or her religion uniquely. How a Buddhist client meditates or a Seventh-day Adventist keeps Sabbath and prays may differ from how another of the same faith approaches these activities.

On the other hand, recommended lifestyles and practices of the world's diverse religions have a surprising degree of similarity. Although nurses need not memorize practices of every religion, it is helpful to understand some practices common to many.

Dietary Practices

Many religions proscribe or recommend certain dietary guidelines. Some encourage vegetarianism (e.g., Buddhist, Hindu, Seventh-day Adventist, Sikhism, Hare Krishna,) and others proscribe pork (e.g., Islam, Judaism). Hindus will not eat beef, considering the cow a sacred creature. Many individuals choose a simple or vegetarian diet as they develop spiritually. A vegetarian diet for some (e.g., New Age) is an ecological statement, while for others it is a way of respecting the body as a "temple of God" or a means to aid spiritual alertness.

Jewish law defines not only what a Jew should eat, but how the food should be prepared and consumed. A kosher diet permits animals that do not have cloven hooves, regurgitate their food, or eat their prey; fish with fins and scales; and chicken, turkey, and duck. Only meat that has been ritually slaughtered is kosher. Kosher requires that meats and dairy products not be cooked or consumed together. A strict observer maintains two sets of cookware and dishes, one for meats and another for dairy products. Observant Jews must wait a specified period between consuming meat and dairy products (it varies from one-half to six hours); they may also rinse their mouth between meals. A very observant Jewish client may not only refuse meat and milk in the same meal but request only fruit or other uncooked items so as to avoid receiving food that was cooked in pans that have contained both meat and dairy products. A practicing Jew may also eat only foods prepared under the supervision of a rabbi. Store-bought foods are labeled to indicate that this kosher certification process has occurred.

Fasting and abstaining from certain foods is often an element of religious practice. During the month of Ramadan, for example, Muslims fast from dawn to sunset. Jews keep a strict fast on Yom Kippur and Tishah B'Ab. Many Christians choose to avoid certain foods during the 40 days prior to Easter. Some Episcopalians avoid meat on Fridays. A short fast (1 to 6 hours) prior to receiving the Eucharist is advocated for Eastern Orthodox and Roman Catholics. While some fasts accompany high holy days, others are observed voluntarily as part of one's devotional practices. Fasting cleanses the body, clears the mind, and fosters spiritual alertness. It is important for nurses to note, however, that religions typically nullify these proscriptions for the sick or any for whom a fast would be unhealthful (e.g., children, pregnant women, diabetics, elderly).

Many religions forbid all use of or strongly discourage abuse of alcohol and drugs (e.g., Buddhist, Islam, Hare Krishna, fundamental and evangelical Christian, Mormon, Seventh-day Adventist). Stimulants like caffeine and nicotine are also discouraged or prohibited in many traditions (e.g., Buddhist, Islam, fundamental Christian denominations, Quaker, Mormon, Seventh-day Adventist). In contrast to these injunctions against intoxicating drink or drugs, some religions approve of the judicious use of wine to complement ceremonies and mind-altering drugs to induce mystical experiences. The mild hallucinogen, peyote, was legally used for some Native American religious rituals before it was ruled illegal by the Supreme Court in 1990. Judaism recognizes wine in nonabusive amounts as a complement to many religious rituals. A sip of wine is often provided during the Christian Eucharist, though several traditions substitute grape juice.

Observing Holy Days

Most religions have weekly and annual holy days. Some Hindus may observe certain religious practices as they worship a god specific to a certain day of the week. Muslims consider Friday their holy day, and will gather for a worship service at noon. Jews, Seventh-day Adventists, and other Sabbatarians observe the seventh day of the week as their Sabbath (from sunset Friday evening to sunset Saturday). Most Christians consider Sunday as the "Lord's Day." Most religions celebrate annual holy days. These annual events may commemorate the birth or death of the founder of the religion or other significant events that occurred during the early history of the religion. Some holy days are observed with somber penitence, and others are met with jubilance and festivity.

If appropriate, the nurse assesses how a client observes a holy day. Weekly holy days are typically times for rest and recreation (physical, social, and especially spiritual). Attending a worship service is a characteristic activity as are special meals and time with family and friends. Observant Sabbath keepers will avoid conducting unnecessary business on their holy day. Orthodox and some Conservative Jews will not drive, turn on electricity, or do a number of proscribed activities. Clients receiving health care on a holy day may request that only minimal or essential procedures be done.

Religious Objects

Clients often carry personal religious items to aid them in their worship or for spiritual comfort. Many religious traditions, for example, encourage the use of prayer beads to focus prayer (e.g., Roman Catholic, Eastern Orthodox, Islam). Fingering a prayer bead, like rubbing a stone, can relieve stress. Amulets and talismans are other religious items a client may cling to during times of distress. Amulets are objects believed to ward off disease and misfortune. Mormon "temple undergarments," worn for protection and to provide modesty, exemplify clothing that functions as an amulet.

The use of talismans, objects considered to bring good fortune and health, is prevalent within many cultures. Such objects are often worn as jewelry (e.g., lockets, pendants), and their removal can create feelings of discomfort in some clients. When removal of religious articles of clothing or jewelry is absolutely necessary (e.g., some surgeries and medical procedures), the client or family members should be consulted about where and how to safely store them.

Other religious items a client may use when a health challenge presents include objects for visual focus like the crucifix or cross (i.e., Christian, especially Roman Catholic), icons or pictures of Christ or a saint (e.g., Roman Catholic, Eastern Orthodox), idol or sculptured image of a god (e.g., Hindu gods, Buddha), or yantras and mandalas (foci for meditation, used within Buddhism, Hinduism, New Age movement). Religious articles of clothing may also be used by a client during prayer or worship (e.g., prayer shawls, caps, or other head coverings, which express deference to God, worn by Jews, Muslims, and others). Items that may be used in religious practices include incense, candles, gongs or bells, and religious books.

Religious books a client might bring into a health care setting include sacred scriptures as well as liturgical, devotional, and prayer books compiled for personal or public worship. A devout religious person may study ancillary texts that provide interpretation or support for that religion's scriptures. A Christian Scientist, for example, may read Mary Baker Eddy's "Science and Health with Key to the Scriptures." A Seventh-day Adventist may read one of Ellen G. White's many books (e.g., "Ministry of Healing" or "Desire of Ages"). A Latter-day Saint may read the "Book of Mormon." Others may want to read prayers from a prayer book (e.g., Episcopal, Eastern Orthodox, Jewish, Lutheran, Roman Catholic). Although many Western religions accept the Bible as sacred scripture, the version that is approved varies. While many religions accept most of the modern translations of the Bible as accurate, others recommend a specific version, such as their own (e.g., Jehovah's Witnesses) or the King James Version (KJV) that uses seventeenth-century English (e.g., Mormon).

Religious Practices Related to Birthing

Some religions (e.g., Judaism, Islam, many Christian traditions) teach that life begins at conception and elective abortion is murder. Roman Catholicism teaches that mechanical and hormonal methods for contraception are also wrong. And nearly every religion forbids sexual intercourse outside of marriage.

While baptist Christian religions (e.g., Baptists, Pentecostal, Mormon, Seventh-day Adventist) believe an individual should be baptized by complete immersion under water when old enough to understand and choose baptism, others believe in infant baptism and baptize by immersion (e.g., some Eastern Orthodox) or sprinkling or placing small amounts of water on the forehead (e.g., Roman Catholic, Episcopal). For fetuses or infants who are born dead or will die soon, a nurse may need to offer a baptism if a chaplain or representative of the clergy is not available and the parents request it.

It may surprise nurses to learn that they can perform an infant baptism. It does not require prior theological training or ordination. It would be respectful, however, if the nurse did share the essential Christian beliefs supporting the practice. The requisite components to an infant baptism include saying "I now baptize you in the name of the Father, the Son, and the Holy Spirit" while sprinkling or touching the infant's forehead with water. For a Greek Orthodox infant whose condition is grave, touch the forehead three times with water (to reflect the trinity) or move the infant in the air in the sign of the cross if immersion might be detrimental. Although the baptism can be as simple as this, the nurse should give thought to other ways to make the ritual special. The infant being baptized, for example, could be dressed in white or special clothing, the parents may hold their child while the baptism is performed, and the nurse may want to add a prayer or read a poem or blessing—or sing a hymn! Understanding the function and ingredients of a meaningful ritual (see Chapter 9) will help a nurse to create a memorable baptism.

For Jews and Muslims, the circumcision of males is a religious practice. Jewish law teaches that circumcision should occur on the eighth day after birth. This ceremony is performed by a religious person who is dedicated to this task. If Jewish or Moslem parents have concerns about circumcision, the nurse can provide information and support their decision.

Religious Practices Related to Healing

Several religions (especially Christian traditions) offer healing services that encourage persons desiring healing to name their concerns, after which a spiritual leader prays for that healing. Some healing practices involve the cleric's anointing the client (e.g., placing a drop of blessed oil on the forehead) and saying a blessing or petitionary prayer for the client. Often, these anointing rituals are requested when clients are perilously ill. Some clients may prefer that such a healing ceremony be enacted privately in their home or hospital room. Some deeply appreciate the nurse's attendance.

The Roman Catholic sacrament "Anointing of the Sick," which was formerly referred to as "Extreme Unction" or "Last Rites" is an example of a healing ritual. Although in the past this mandatory Roman Catholic sacrament was performed just prior to death, it is now offered for all who are sick. Some Roman Catholics, however, may not understand this and mis-construe a nurse's offer to call a priest or say a prayer as an indication that death is imminent.

A theme of nineteenth-century American Christianity reflected in nursing literature of the era was "cleanliness is next to Godliness." In several religious traditions, the fact that cleanliness is highly valued manifests in various ways. A Hindu, for example, may request that a ritual be performed to cleanse a hospital room of evil spirits before being admitted to it. An orthodox Jewish woman will go to a mikveh (a bath) seven days after the cessation of any uterine bleeding (e.g., menses) or prior to resuming sexual relations, completely submerge herself in this bath, and say a blessing. Some orthodox men will also go to a mikveh to ritually cleanse themselves prior to a holy day. Christian baptism by immersion, likewise, symbolizes spiritual cleansing. The parallel between a nurse's ritual of bathing a client and a religious ritual of cleansing should be noted. The nurse bathing a client can offer more than physical cleansing. This nursing ritual, frequently relegated to unlicensed personnel, provides an opportunity for demonstrating caring in an emotional and spiritual way.

Religious Practices Related to Dying and Bereavement

Religious beliefs influence how people mourn. Many faiths share a belief in an afterlife. Hindus and Buddhists believe they will be reincarnated into another being, while most Christians and Muslims believe there will be a resurrection for the dead, a final Judgment, and an afterlife for each person in heaven or hell. Several traditions (i.e., Muslim, Jewish, Hindu) encourage family members to wash the deceased's body immediately after the death and cover it with a white sheet. Deceased Jews may be prepared for burial by a Jewish burial society. Recommendations for a hasty and simple burial are offered by some religions. A Muslim, for example, is to be buried preferably on the same day as the death, and a Jew as soon as possible after death. While some religions prefer cremation (e.g., Buddhist, Hindu, Hare Krishna, Sikh), others encourage burial of the body (e.g, Baha'i, Islam, some Jews, Mormon). Jews show additional respect for the dead by keeping a vigil with the body until it is interred. Others believe respect for the dead requires that organ donation and autopsies be avoided (e.g., some Jews, Christian Science, Muslim).

Inherent in all religions is respect for the sacredness of life. How this principle guides ethical decisions about when to prolong or sustain life varies. While many religions oppose active euthanasia (using direct intervention to cause death), the arguments for and against passive euthanasia (allowing death by withholding or withdrawing life-sustaining care) are complex. It is important for nurses to recognize that many clients struggle to reconcile respect for life with the desire to end suffering that appears to be meaningless or to begin the afterlife (e.g., "die and go to heaven").

Mourning practices are also influenced by religious traditions. These traditions help determine if a religious leader is to be called for prayer at the time of the death, how the funeral or memorial occurs, and how the mourners grieve afterwards. The Jewish tradition, for example, encourages mourners to fully express sad emotions. The simple wooden casket remains closed. At the burial, the family throws dirt on the casket. Afterwards, the family is socially supported. Friends visit and bring food to the home of the grieving family while they "sit shiva" for seven days after the burial.

Worship Practices

Worship includes private or devotional as well as public or communal practices. Communal worship typically occurs at shrines, temples, mosques, synagogues, and churches. Sometimes, when there are not enough believers to support such a public venue, believers will gather together in a home or other informal setting. For most clients, the social support inherent in communal worship is an important aspect of religion. The inability to attend religious services may signify the loss of feeling part of a spiritual community and a change in the accustomed way of experiencing the Divine. Clients may verbalize this loss with statements like, "I miss the music at church" or "I miss the gathering time after services."

Personal approaches to worship reflect individual needs. Individuals may have a set time each day that they dedicate to devotional reading or some form of prayer (e.g., singing, writing, or meditating during prayer). A client may spend a half hour each morning reading the Bible and keeping a prayer journal, and another may take 20 minutes twice a day to light a candle and meditate. Regardless of the activities a client's personal worship entails, a nurse will want to facilitate by ensuring quiet, uninterrupted privacy and by providing physical comfort measures beforehand that facilitate relaxed concentration. For example, a client receiving narcotics who wants to spend time in meditative prayer may want to time the administration and dose of the narcotic so it will minimally interfere with consciousness.

Box 10-2 summarizes key aspects of major faith traditions.

Box 10-2. Guide to Major Faith Traditions

Buddhism

Title Used to Address Deity/Clergy	No deity; however, some relate to Buddha (or a lesser Buddha) like a god Monks and priests (whose primary role is teaching)
Prayer/Worship Considerations	Meditation; some may petition Buddha May go to temple or shrine to offer prayers and gifts to Buddha or monks; may have shrine at home
Beliefs About Afterlife	Reincarnation until Nirvana is attained
Guidelines for Diet—Use of Alcohol and Drugs	Some are vegetarian Discouraged

Health Care Implications (Buddhism)

- Cleanliness is highly valued, evidenced by practices such as removing footwear and gargling.
- Meaning attributed to suffering may affect use of pain management strategies.
- Physical illness or suffering is inevitable as well as an opportunity for transformation.
- Physical disease results from good or bad karma (result of acts previously committed).
- May make pilgrimages to a shrine or buddha of healing to seek healing.
- Some Buddhist monks offer healing practices (e.g., invocations, breathing exercises, massage, herbs).
- May request priest to chant when death is imminent.
- Intense grieving is considered inappropriate.
- Suicide is forbidden except for self-sacrifice for religious reasons.

(continues)

Box 10-2. Guide to Major Faith Traditions *(continued)*

Christianity

Title Used to Address Deity/Clergy	God, Lord, Savior, and other descriptors; Trinity comprised of Father, Son (i.e., Jesus Christ), and Holy Spirit; many address saints (Roman Catholic, Episcopal, and Orthodox) Priest or Father (Roman Catholic, Episcopal, and Orthodox); Reverend or minister (traditional mainline Protestants); Pastor or minister (evangelical and fundamentalist); Elder (Jehovah's Witnesses, Mormon)
Prayer/Worship Considerations	Most use conversational and petitionary styles; Roman Catholic, Orthodox, Episcopal, and some others often use written or memorized prayers Many attend church on Sunday (Seventh-day Adventists on Saturday); many participate in private prayer or devotional time daily
Beliefs About Afterlife	Most believe in final judgment that determines heaven or hell
Guidelines for Diet—Use of Alcohol and Drugs	Many avoid certain foods during Lent and fast before taking communion; Seventh-day Adventists usually vegetarian Discouraged especially by fundamentalists, evangelicals, Mormons, and Seventh-day Adventists

Box 10-2. Guide to Major Faith Traditions *(continued)*

Health Care Implications (Christianity)

- Jehovah's Witnesses refuse most blood products.

- Christian Scientists refuse many medical interventions and prefer to see their own practitioners.

- Many Christians request Communion when unable to attend religious services.

- May refrain from unnecessary medical procedures on the "Lord's Day" (Sunday) or Sabbath (Saturday).

- May receive care from a religious healer (e.g, Christian Science practitioner, faith healer).

- May request a priest or minister to receive their confession.

- Mormon may request a blessing which is performed by two Mormon men

(continues)

Box 10-2. Guide to Major Faith Traditions *(continued)*

Hinduism

Title Used to Address Deity/Clergy	Brahman, Vishnu, Shiva (the trinity); Durga (feminine form of God); also worship other incarnations of these gods Gurus, swamis are teachers of religion and holy men
Prayer/Worship Considerations	Many have daily meditation at shrine at home; yoga May visit shrine on annual holy days; use of image of a god and other objects that focus meditation
Beliefs About Afterlife	Reincarnation
Guidelines for Diet—Use of Alcohol and Drugs	Many are vegetarian; most eat no beef Many avoid all use

Health Care Implications (Hinduism)

- Cleanliness is very important.
- Health results when body elements are balanced by consuming food and drink in the right way, amount, and time.
- Prefer foods fresh or cooked in oil that observe Ayurvedic theory that recommends foods achieve a balance of tastes (e.g., sweet, sour, bitter, salty), and heating and cooling effects.
- Attribute disease to multiple factors (e.g., biological infection, deity's displeasure, disharmonious relationships, karma, eating the wrong food).
- Prefer cremation soon after death.
- At death, water is poured into mouth; family washes the body.

Box 10-2. Guide to Major Faith Traditions *(continued)*

Islam

Title Used to Address Deity/Clergy	Allah (Arabic for God) Imam (lay religious leader)
Prayer/Worship Considerations	Ritual prayers five times per day with ablutions prior Attend mosque or gather with group at noon Fridays
Beliefs About Afterlife	Resurrection of the dead and final judgment; heaven or hell
Guidelines for Diet—Use of Alcohol and Drugs	No pork Strongly discouraged

Health Care Implications (Islam)

- Avoid male clinicians to care for female clients and vice versa.
- Nakedness considered shameful. Muslim woman may require husband's permission to undress for a male health care professional.
- Fetus considered a complete human being; babies traditionally breastfeed for 2 years.
- Children, elderly, pregnant, or sick Muslims exempt from fasting during Ramadan.
- Bride's virginity a matter of honor for entire family; medical procedures that may tear hymen need to be documented in order to support proof of virginity to a future husband.
- Washing corpse is one of numerous prescriptions for postmortem care; burial occurs immediately; only men may attend funerals.

Box 10-2. Guide to Major Faith Traditions *(concluded)*

Judaism

Title Used to Address Deity/Clergy	God (written with respect as G-d or YHWH; spoken terms include Lord, the Holy One, Adonai, and other Hebrew words) Rabbi (who has received extensive education)
Prayer/Worship Considerations	Prayers from prayer book, privately and during religious rituals Attend synagogue Saturdays(Shabbat); possibly on Friday evening and annual holy days
Beliefs About Afterlife	No official stance on existence of an afterlife
Guidelines for Diet—Use of Alcohol and Drugs	Varying degrees of observance of kosher dietary rules (e.g., do not mix dairy and meat, no pork or shellfish) Wine in nonintoxicating amounts often part of religious ritual

Health Care Implications (Judaism)

- Heath care decisions reflect mandate to respect and preserve life.
- Believe God created the body; it is on loan for the duration of life; physical happiness is to be enjoyed.
- May decline unnecessary health care procedures on Shabbat.
- Sabbath observance may require not writing, traveling in vehicles, turning on lights, stove, or other electrical appliance.
- Orthodox and some Conservative men wear a kippah or yarmulka (skull cap) to show deference to God; a tallit (fringed prayer shawl) and tefillin (two small black leather boxes containing Scripture) are worn by Jewish men during daily morning worship.
- Sickness and suffering explained by sin, physical and psychological causes; some may explain it with demons.
- Cremation forbidden; burial in wooden casket as soon as possible after death encouraged.

NURSING IMPLICATIONS

A cursory knowledge of religious practices provides an awareness and sensitivity to the breadth of possible religious practices used by clients. With this awareness, nurses can further assess for specific practices when appropriate. A Jewish family of a dying client, for example, can be asked what religious practices they would like to observe at the time of death. Or a Muslim who is being admitted to a hospital can be queried regarding if and how he or she would like a nurse to facilitate the daily prayers. The nurse's ability to model comfort with talking about religious practices will encourage the client to feel comfortable describing personal religiosity.

Some clients will welcome a nurse's queries about their religion. Others may be embarrassed or irritated. Some clients view their religious practices as private and not for a nurse to "meddle with." Ethical spiritual care requires the nurse to respect client responses. Because religion is such an intimate experience and some clients are very private people, the nurse should not be surprised if a client declines an offer of assistance with religious practice. An appropriate response might be, "That's fine. Please know that if you do find yourself needing some assistance with practicing your religion, that I am willing to help if I can."

For some clients, a health challenge can precipitate an increased interest in religion or more faithful adherence to practices. It is possible that a client may desire to begin certain religious practices, but feel unable to because of a lack of experience or knowledge. A seriously ill client, for example, may want to pray but may feel she does not "know how to do it." A nurse may be able to provide some guidance but may also need to make a referral to a spiritual care expert.

Addressing Nurse–Client Religious Conflict

A nurse's religious orientation often differs from that of a client, and sometimes a client's religious practices may clash with those of the nurse. A hemorrhaging Jehovah's Witness, for example, may refuse a blood transfusion for religious reasons. (For Jehovah's Witnesses, being given blood is considered "medical rape.") A Christian Scientist may refuse immunization for his child. An immigrant from South America may want her shaman to exorcise evil spirits by blowing smoke over her face or washing her body with a hallucinogenic plant solution. Practices that may conflict with Western health care practice often create ethical dilemmas.

It is possible to develop approaches to healing that will be acceptable to the client and nurse whose religious orientations differ. A clergyperson or an informed representative of the client's religion may be able to provide guidance. Often, lay members are not clear about religious rules or rationales. Jehovah's Witnesses, for example, have representatives available to discuss the choice to refuse blood transfusions. These representatives can clarify which blood by-products are unacceptable and which are permitted and provide resources and ideas about how to manage the situation (e.g., provide information about physicians who perform blood-sparing surgeries or use alternative techniques to manage anemia). Careful listening to clients and their religious representatives and examination of personal religious attitudes can assist nurses to provide ethical care to clients whose beliefs differ from their own. Box 10-3 illustrates a nursing approach that incorporates respect for client religious practices.

Although it is often possible to create a strategy that will be acceptable to both client and nurse, occasionally these conflicts are not resolved in a manner that is comfortable for the nurse. Ethical care requires the nurse to respect the client's religiosity and the needs that arise from it even when doing so may contribute to an outcome that the nurse may consider detrimental. The nurse may draw comfort in such situations by recognizing that the outcome was one that was desired by the client and was likely perceived as ultimately appropriate and spiritually helpful. Consider a woman who is a Jehovah's Witness and refuses a lifesaving blood transfusion, resulting in her death. Although her death may represent a negative outcome from the nurse's perspective, the client's perspective deserves consideration. For this client, perhaps what matters most is being able to avoid "medical rape" by refusing procedures that to her signify spiritual disobedience and to receive support to live and die in harmony with her understanding of God's commands.

The line that separates espousing religious beliefs that conflict with traditional Western health care practices from those that are destructive toward self or others is not always clear. For example, are Christian Science parents harming their daughter when they refuse medical therapies to treat her life-threatening illness? Is the man with a bipolar disorder who, for religious reasons, feels admonished to fast for an extended period harming himself? Because it may sometimes be difficult to determine the ethically appropriate approach in such situations, it is imperative that nurses document thoroughly and consult or convene the relevant parties. Not only do the client and family need to discuss the meaning and application of religious beliefs with health care team members, but the health

Box 10-3. One Nurse's Story: Respecting Client Religious Beliefs

Roughly three days after giving birth, a mother's breasts will engorge with milk. If the milk is not extracted adequately, milk stasis will cause discomfort and possibly mastitis. Typical nursing interventions for alleviating engorgement include applying heat and pumping (with an electric pump or manually).

These interventions can be problematic for the orthodox Jewish mother who keeps Shabbat from Friday sundown to Saturday sundown. Rabbinic Law prohibits threshing, grinding, igniting a fire, building, and other work activities on the Sabbath. This law would be violated if a woman were to manually pump milk with the purpose of storing it or use an electric pump, because using electricity is viewed as lighting a fire. Taking a warm shower, massaging the breasts with lotion, and taking medication also violate the Rabbinic Law, which does, however, encourage breastfeeding.

Israeli nurse Ilana Chertok's (1999) study of Jewish law led her to identify helpful options that are permitted for a mother with engorged breasts. These included: manually expressing the milk into a container with salt or soap to render it unusable, massaging the breasts without lotion, applying a warm water bottle with water heated prior to the start of the Sabbath, using cold compresses that do not require wringing to make (e.g., package of frozen vegetables), applying cabbage leaves (which contain the edema-decreasing enzyme sinigrin), and using an electric pump but not pumping more than 17 mL at one time.

For nurses who are non-Orthodox Jews, followers of other faiths, or nonreligious, these proscriptions may seem ludicrous. Yet what may appear incredible to an outsider, is nevertheless credible, meaningful, and an accepted part of life for the insider who demonstrates respect to God, ancestors, family, and values through such practices.

Issues such as those presented above can challenge the nurse's customary approaches to providing care. Chertok's creativity demonstrates how the nurse can explore alternatives when challenges presented by the client's religious background arise. Whether or not they agree with a client's refusal of certain medical treatments or use of unusual healing techniques, nurses must develop responses that are ethically and spiritually nurturing.

care team may also need to consult religious, legal, and medical ethics experts.

Harmful Religiosity: How to Care

How does the nurse attend to the spiritual needs of clients whose religious beliefs may lead to a harmful effect? The following practice guidelines are suggested:

- Avoid jumping to conclusions about the potential harmfulness of a client's religion. A thorough spiritual assessment is required in order to support this conclusion. Be aware of any personal biases about religiosity while conducting the assessment.
- Refer clients to a trained chaplain or a psychologist sensitive to religious issues (see Chapter 4). If a client's religiosity is determined to be delusional or compulsive, bringing in the client's spiritual leader to openly discuss unhealthful views can also be helpful (Greenberg & Witztum, 1991).
- Miles (1996) offered some specific questions for helping clients to think about potentially harmful religious beliefs, including:
  - " 'Do you believe that God requires people to suffer as atonement for their sins?'
  - 'What does God gain from our suffering?'
  - 'Do you think God asks this of everyone in pain?'
  - 'What makes you different from others in the eyes of God?'
  - 'How does this belief fit with your image of a loving God?' "
    (p. 47).
- Some clients view God as a rescuer who performs miracles by suspending the laws of nature. Skilled spiritual caregivers can assist these clients to "reimagine" God in a broader way (Connors & Smith, 1996). Connors and Smith argue that holding a narrow image of God does injustice both to the mysteries of God and human experiences (i.e., health, sickness, life, death). Clients who are willing to explore other scriptural images of God may benefit. Connors and Smith offer two examples of religious reimagination: (1) viewing God as Emmanuel (present One) instead of as rescuer and (2) learning to perceive the ability to accept tragedy or feel the loving presence of others (rather than the cure for a disease) as a miracle.

- Recognize and manage personal emotional responses. Kumasaka (1996) recounted how her inner turmoil over the need to rescue a client in pain, who for religious reasons refused medications, was her own problem rather than her client's. Even though Kumasaka understood that ethical, client-centered nursing care required her to allow her client to suffer in pain, she still struggled with feelings of guilt.

KEY POINTS

- Religious beliefs influence how clients interpret many life experiences, including illness and death, as well as how they care for their personal health. Conversely, health challenges and medical treatments may affect the client's ability to practice religion.

- Numerous empirical studies have demonstrated positive relationships between religiosity and physical and mental health.

- Levin (1994) hypothesized several mechanisms that may explain the health benefits of religiosity. These include: behavior; psychosocial effects; the psychodynamics of beliefs, religious rites, and faith; a superempirical force.

- Major faith traditions include Hinduism, Buddhism, Judaism, Christianity, and Islam. Syncretistic religions, such as Sikhism, Baha'i, and Nation of Islam, have developed subsequently and reflect some of the beliefs and practices of these major religions.

- When offering to facilitate religious practices, the nurse respects the client's wishes and manages differences with sensitivity.

- Unique and salient religious beliefs and practices found across many different faith traditions include:
  - Weekly holy days or Sabbaths when persons attend religious services, enjoy their families, and often refrain from necessary work.
  - Use of religious objects and worship practices to commune with higher spiritual beings or a deity.

- Solemn and festive annual holy days that commemorate an important historical event significant to the religious tradition.
- Afterlife in some form (e.g., heaven or hell, reincarnation).
- Prohibition of actions that are considered disrespectful of the sanctity of life (e.g., elective abortion and active euthanasia).
- Vegetarianism and abstention from pork or certain other meats.

LOOK WITHIN TO LEARN

1. Sometimes, the word *religious* is used to describe the fervor and devotion of one's approach to a nonreligious endeavor. "He watches football religiously every Monday night" is an example. What activities in your life might your friends or family say you approach religiously? By engaging in these activities, in what ways might it be said that you are demonstrating a spiritual desire—a yearning or thirst for a meaningful experience?

2. Scholars have theorized that there are two kinds of religiosity: intrinsic (in which religion is a framework that provides meaningfulness) and extrinsic (in which religion is a social tool for self-serving purposes). If you are religious, how would you rate yourself on a scale of 1 (very intrinsic) to 5 (very extrinsic)?

3. How congruent are your religious practices with your religious beliefs? How might any incongruencies between your beliefs and practices affect your response to a religious client? In what other ways might your own religiosity (or nonreligiosity) influence your response to a client's?

REFERENCES

Bold print indicates those that are most recommended.

Allan, J. (1994). The spiritual search. In *Eerdman's handbook to the world's religions*. Grand Rapids, MI: Eerdmans.

Burnard, P. (1988). The spiritual needs of atheists and agnostics. *The Professional Nurse, 4*(3), 130, 132.

Chertok, I. (1999). Relief of breast engorgement for the Sabbath-observant Jewish woman. *Journal of Obstetric, Gynecologic, and Neonatal Nursing, 28*, 365–369.

Connors, R. B., Jr., & Smith, M. L. (1996). Religious insistence on medical treatment: Christian theology and re-imagination. *Hastings Center Report, 26*(4): 23–30.

Deloria, V., Jr. (1994). *God is red: A native view of religion*. Golden, CO: Fulcrum.

Doyne, N. (1990). Channeling and other esoteric methods of self-care. *Holistic Nursing Practice, 4*(4), 70–76.

Gallup, G. H., Jr. (1996). *Religion in America*. Princeton, NJ: Princeton Religion Research Center.

Gartner, J., Larson, D. B., & Allen, G. D. (1991). Religious commitment and mental health: A review of the empirical literature. *Journal of Psychology and Theology, 19*(1), 6–25.

Greenberg, D., & Witztum, E. (1991). Problems in the treatment of religious patients. *American Journal of Psychotherapy, 45*, 554–565.

Hufford, D. J. (1993). Epistemologies in religious healing. *The Journal of Medicine and Philosophy, 18*, 175–194.

Hupcey, J. E. (2000). Feeling safe: The psychosocial needs of ICU patients. *Journal of Nursing Scholarship, 32*(4), 361–367.

Jarvis, G. K., & Northcott, H. C. (1987). Religion and differences in morbidity and mortality. *Social Science and Medicine, 25*, 813–824.

Koenig, H. G. (1997). *Is religion good for your health? The effects of religion on physical and mental health*. New York: The Hawarth Press.

Kumasaka, L. (1996). "My pain is God's will": A pain management nurse's dilemma. *American Journal of Nursing, 96*(6), 45–46.

Larson, D. B., Sherrill, K. A., Lyons, J. S., Craigie, F. C., Thielman, S. B., Greenwold, M. A., & Larson, S. S. (1992). Associations between dimensions of religious commitment and mental health reported in the *American Journal of Psychiatry* and *Archives of General Psychiatry*: 1978–1989. *American Journal of Psychiatry, 149*, 557–559.

Levin, J. S. (1994). Religion and health: Is there an association, is it valid, and is it causal? *Social Science and Medicine, 38*, 1475–1482.

Levin, J. S., & Schiller, P. L. (1987). Is there a religious factor in health? *Journal of Religion and Health, 26*(1), 9–36.

Matthews, D. A., McCullough, M. E., Larson, D. B., Koenig, H. G., Swyers, J. P., & Milano, M. G. (1998). Religious commitment and health status: A review of the research and implications for family medicine. *Archives of Family Medicine, 7*(2), 118–124.

Miles, A. (1996). "My pain is God's will": A chaplain's perspective. *American Journal of Nursing, 96*(6), 47.

Numbers, R. L., & Amundsen, D. W. (1986). *Caring and curing: Health and medicine in the Western religious traditions*. New York: Macmillan.

Pargament, K. I. (1997). *The psychology of religion and coping*. New York: Guilford.

Sullivan, L. E. (Ed.). (1989). *Healing and restoring: Health and medicine in the world's religious traditions*. New York: Macmillan.

Taylor, E. J., Highfield, M. F., & Amenta, M. O. (1994). Attitudes and beliefs regarding spiritual care: A survey of cancer nurses. *Cancer Nursing, 17*(6), 479–487.

11

Nurturing Spirituality

Providing spiritual care incorporates a way of *being* and a way of *being with* a client. Although this text has admonished, "Don't just do something, be there!," the nurse can *do* a number of things to promote client spiritual health. This chapter introduces a variety of spirit-nurturing activities as nursing interventions for clients. These activities may also benefit nurses who seek to explore their own spirituality.

NATURE: ENGAGING THE SPIRIT

Many religious traditions consider nature, or the outdoors and its world of living things, to be the handiwork or a literal illustration of God. Some worldviews see spiritual entities as housed within nature, or that nature is the embodiment of God. Regardless of orientation, many people feel that experiencing aspects of the natural environment—a deserted beach, a shimmering wheat field, a majestic mountain, a lush forest, or a quiet stream—may feel like a spiritual experience.

Nature's Healing Effects

Although their samples were small, two qualitative studies conducted by nurse researchers provide initial evidence that hospitalized clients value the act of contemplating nature and consider it to aid their spiritual health and mental focus (Narayanasamy, 1995; Travis & McAuley, 1998). Evidence also suggests that viewing nature contributes to better health outcomes. Travis and McAuley reviewed research that examines the impact of a window view for those who are institutionalized. When a view of natural surroundings was compared with one of an urban scene, research findings associated the natural view with decreased postoperative hospital stay and fewer analgesic requests among surgical patients, decreased need for health care services among prison inmates, and decreased ailments and headaches and increased job satisfaction among office workers.

Natural environments are believed to have meditative effects that provide "access to our higher self" (Cumes, 1998, p. 79). Cumes created a helpful analogy for understanding this process of drawing from nature to gain self- and spiritual awareness: "The process that occurs with prolonged exposure to the wilderness is very much like peeling away the layers of an onion to get to its core—with Self being at the center. This peeling process can lead to self-awareness, peak experiences, and moments of transcendence ('wilderness rapture')" (p. 85). Cumes, summarizing research findings about responses to wilderness environments, indicates that this kind of setting contributes to:

- Increased self-awareness or "being more like myself"
- Feelings of awe, wonder, and oneness
- Humility, recognition that human control over nature is an illusion
- Increased thoughtfulness and receptivity to others
- A greater sense of living simply and in the present moment
- Increased mindfulness and focus
- A sense of vigor and renewal
- Relief from addictive urges
- Appreciation for solitude

Ruffing's (1997) findings from in-depth interviews with 24 Christians corroborate the spiritually beneficial effect of being in a natural setting. Ruffing observed several characteristics of mystical nature experiences described by interviewees. Natural surroundings:

- Fostered reconnection with self physically, emotionally, and spiritually. Interviewees felt more whole and more attuned to their deepest, real selves.
- Provided perspective to problems, increasing their awareness of being a part of something larger.
- Enhanced relationships. Communion in the nonhuman world of nature correlated with a sense of community among people.
- Made them feel closer to God. They perceived a Creator Spirit as disclosing its intimate, ordering, and caring presence.

Implications for Nursing Practice

These research findings suggest that helping a client to experience nature promotes spiritual as well as other dimensions of health. When clients are confined to home, hospital, or community setting, nurses need to be creative about how to encourage them to experience nature or how to bring nature to them. Box 11-1 relates the experience of a nurse whose creativity helped her to facilitate a positive connection with nature for a dying client.

Box 11-1. One Nurse's Story: The Anointing

At the time of the following incident, Wendy Stiver, RN, BSN, MA, was working in an inpatient oncology unit at a community hospital.

When we think of providing spiritual care for our patients, some obvious interventions come to mind: prayer, offering communion, laying on of hands, chanting, and so on. But just as spirituality is a part of each person's uniqueness, our interventions may be equally unique. Sometimes providing spiritual care means going out in the rain and getting cold and wet.

Box 11-1. One Nurse's Story: The Anointing *(continued)*

I was caring for Mary, a woman with end-stage peritoneal cancer. She had fought a long, valiant battle and had now come close to her last day. We did the usual things: kept her linens clean and dry, started a morphine drip, positioned her edematous body as comfortably as we could, and turned her so she could look out the window at the nearby mountains. We brought the family coffee and tea, set up a cot in the room, and provided round-the-clock hugs and tissues. We ignored visiting hours and rules about children sitting on beds.

One day we had one of those seemingly endless winter rainstorms. Our unit had large windows, so patients witnessed the storm in all its glory. One of Mary's last wishes before slipping off into a coma was to go out in the rain one more time.

As afternoon approached and her death appeared imminent, some of the nurses and rehabilitation staff decided to take Mary out in the rain. We weren't quite sure how to do this, because she was a large, immobile woman on a pressure-reducing mattress, receiving oxygen and intravenous drugs and fluids. We also chose to disregard the fact that she was on the fourth floor. The "hows" weren't important—Mary was going out in the rain.

After much strategizing, four of us went to Mary's room, where one of her devoted nieces was keeping vigil. Mary was unresponsive, but I was confident that she would know—and welcome—what we were doing. With the niece's approval, we unplugged the bed, the oxygen, the pumps and poles, and the bed alarms, and started moving Mary in her bed down the hallway.

A choir of conversation erupted among us. It went something like this:

"Where are we going?"

"To the fire escape landing."

"We can't do that!"

"Yes, we can."

"The bed won't fit through the door!"

(continues)

Box 11-1. One Nurse's Story: The Anointing *(concluded)*

"We'll take off the rails if we have to."

"The door alarm will go off!"

"I'll go hold it down at the desk."

"We can't get the bed over the door jamb—it's too high to get wheelchairs over, let alone this heavy bed."

"Push harder! Woman-power can do anything!"

"You're crazy!"

"Yes."

"It's raining!"

"That's the point."

The more we struggled, the more determined we became. After much grunting, we got Mary in her bed out on the landing, in the fresh, cold December air. "Mary, you're out in the rain!" cried her niece.

Mary's eyes opened wide and her face brightened. Her niece sprinkled Mary with rainwater. Then together, we anointed Mary with nature's holy water. We blessed her, each in our own silent way, and watched her relax back into unresponsiveness.

There we stood: a mix of faiths and skill levels, nursing and non-nursing staff. We were gathered together on a fire landing in the cold rain. Some of us were crying, others were smiling, and some were doing both. All of us were wet and cold and knew we'd have to stay in wet clothes for the rest of the shift. It didn't matter. We knew that we'd given Mary an important gift by ministering to the spirit within her that wanted to go out in the rain one more time.

Such acts of spiritual care are truly sacraments of healing: healing for the one who is leaving and healing for those who stay behind. As nurses, we may not think of what we do from a theological perspective, but we do serve as instruments of God's compassion.

Our uniforms allow us to pass through the boundaries of social convention. We are privileged to share some of the most intimate moments in life with total strangers. In these moments, we walk in sacred space and participate in holy acts. Sometimes, that means going out in the rain and getting wet.

Nursing approaches that tap nature as a resource are unlimited and may include:

- Advocating for window views of natural surroundings when there is a choice in patient room assignments or when an institution is being designed or remodeled
- Having flower boxes in a client's room or on a unit
- Bringing wildflowers to a client
- Setting up a fish tank
- Providing access to a pet therapy program
- Showing audiovisuals of nature
- Encouraging family or friends to take the client to a place of natural beauty
- Displaying photographs, illustrations, or murals that depict natural beauty

However a client chooses to experience nature, the nurse should be mindful of the sacredness with which a client might approach this experience. Natural surroundings may evoke rudimentary forms of meditation with the Creator (Ruffing, 1997). The ways in which people experience nature often reflect how they relate to the Divine. What constitutes prayer and an experience of a higher presence is not necessarily expressed in "God language." Some define a spiritual experience simply as the sense of reverence and mystery that results from encountering nature.

Ruffing (1997) observed that elements of nature sometimes provide personal images of God that are comforting during stressful times. A client, for example, may draw courage from viewing a rainbow. Cultivating hyacinths in a flower box may provide metaphorical lessons about spiritual growth as well as delight with their fragrance and beauty.

Cumes (1998) warned that "reentry depression" can occur after a person has experienced "wilderness rapture." Those who experience spiritual euphoria from prolonged exposure to a wilderness setting typically feel some degree of emotional letdown when they leave. Although many clients for whom nurses care may be incapable of pursuing a genuine wilderness experience, a client who is removed from natural surroundings may similarly feel some degree of sadness. The hospitalized client whose room has no outdoor view, for example, may experience sadness upon having to return to her room after a brief outing to an atrium or outdoor patio. Offering a sensitive comment or encouraging the client to take a small, transportable token of nature back to the room may ease melancholy. A client taken in his wheelchair to a garden may be encouraged to retrieve a pebble, a fallen leaf, or flower petal to remember the experience.

STORYTELLING: LISTENING TO THE SPIRIT

Encouraging client storytelling (including life reviews, reminiscence, and oral histories) is a spiritual care intervention that nurtures the spirit in several ways (Banks-Wallace, 1998; Kelly, 1995; Taylor, 1997). Stories allow people to merge seemingly disconnected events into a whole, make sense of them, and gain perspective. Churchill and Churchill (1982) described storytelling as "the forward movement of description of actions and events which makes possible the backward action of self-understanding" (p. 73). Storytelling is also a way of connecting with others, a concrete way to give and receive love. Stories also provide a mechanism for transmitting values and sharing in a way that leaves a legacy. When people tell a story, they transmit meanings that they ascribe to life experiences. To facilitate storytelling, therefore, is to support the process of meaning making, self-understanding, and connecting to others—all of which address spiritual needs.

Storytelling's Healing Effects

When they studied the effects of engaging in storytelling, Rybarczyk and Bellg (1997) found significant reductions in anxiety levels among study participants. They identified five types of reminiscence that reflect the functions of storytelling:

1. *Simple reminiscence* is the act of recalling a past event to elicit positive feelings, find common ground with the listener, and communicate to the listener who the teller is.
2. *Mastery reminiscence* allows storytellers to review ways in which they have mastered past life challenges, thereby helping them to cope with present or future challenges.
3. *Integrative reminiscence* is especially important for those facing a critical juncture or the end of their life. Such reminiscence benefits coping by "connecting the present self to the past self" (p. 17). It allows storytellers to integrate and edit the story of their life, placing it within a larger context.

4. *Transmissive reminiscence* involves recounting previous life events in a way that teaches subsequent generations. Rybarczyk and Bellg suggest that transmissive reminiscence should not be emphasized in health care contexts, because it functions less than other forms in making meaning.

5. *Negative reminiscence*, such as obsessive rumination about an unfortunate event, is less likely to have a therapeutic effect. Although there is benefit in communicating about negative experiences, clients who fixate on them may be candidates for referral.

Implications for Nursing Practice

Among others, Pickrel (1989) and Brady (1999) have suggested strategies for evoking life review storytelling for persons facing death. Although intended for terminally ill clients, these strategies could be adapted for use in a wide range of care situations. Structured activities to encourage a life review include using a set of questions focusing on a specific topic to create an oral history, having the client write or tape an autobiography, creating a family tree or genogram to document facts about one's relations, and drawing a life line or "peaks and valleys" line that shows significant events chronologically. Crafts or other artistic expressions can also be used to tell one's life story (e.g., creating a scrapbook, collage, or song, or designing a monument or shield to depict one's life).

A client may also interact with family to construct a sense of wholeness about the life lived. Activities that help include looking at family treasures and memorabilia—"reminiscentia," inviting family members to share significant stories in person or via mail, attending family reunions, and making a pilgrimage to a place important to family history.

The nurse encourages clients to share anecdotes and reveal more about themselves by asking questions such as:

- What was your life's work about?
- Where were you when [a significant event occurred]?
- When you were a child, what was your favorite toy/game/activity?
- If you had three wishes, what would be the most urgent one to fulfill?

Rybarczyk and Bellg (1997), who developed a program for training volunteer story listeners, identified techniques for promoting effective storytelling and listening. These psychologists suggested that before the client encounter, listeners prepare a set of semistructured interview questions. They also recommended that the guided interview be balanced with spontaneity. As time permits, the listener can coax the teller to describe in more detail, evoking multiple senses, certain parts of the story. The listener should also focus on the positive aspects of a life story, guide the teller to emphasize personal experiences, and encourage reflection. Continual rehashing of an old story is not necessarily helpful; asking creative questions can help the storyteller find enthusiasm and insight in the retelling.

Taylor (1997) developed guidelines for nurses to consider when receiving a client's story, including:

- Remember that storytelling cannot occur, let alone support healing, if there is no story listener. Brody (1987) noted that psychiatry can be summarized as "Chief complaint: No one will listen to my story." Nurses are often bombarded with stories (e.g., illness stories, family stories, anecdotes from daily life). Awareness of the spiritually healing effects of storytelling promotes receptivity to client stories.
- If clients repeat their story, be patient. Repetition may indicate that the teller has been unable to make sense of these life events or that perspective on them has changed. Excessive fixation on a story of misfortune, however, may indicate a need for referral.
- Help clients connect their stories to the present (e.g., "I sense that this story from your childhood is relevant for you now, because . . ." or "I've learned from your story that you highly value . . ., how does this help you now?").
- Perform a story check to help a client increase self-understanding (e.g., "How is this story a metaphor or lesson for your life?" "The stories that you've been telling me seem to have a theme of . . . [identify theme]. Can you tell me more about that?").
- Help clients position their story within a purposeful or redeeming context. Although nurses cannot change a client's story, they can assist clients to cognitively reframe their account so that it is more meaningful. The nurse might respond with questions such as: "This is your life story so far—now how would you like the rest of the story to be?" or "You've had lots of difficult challenges to surmount during your life. What good things have come from these experiences?" or "How has what has happened to you helped to shape who you are today?"

- Remember that how clients tell a story reflects not only what they choose to recollect, but also how they want to be perceived by the listener. Internal questions that can help the nurse understand a client include, "How does this client view him or herself?" "How does this client want me to view him/her?" and "How self-accepting or self-deceiving is this storyteller?"
- Appreciate that though there is likely a counter story, there is no need to discuss it if it will not help the client or the therapeutic relationship.
- To understand meaning embedded in a story, the nurse can apply analytical reasoning while listening to the story. Questions that guide this story analysis are presented in Box 11-2.

Not every client can tell a story cogently. Those with advanced dementia, for example, may be unable to express their stories in ways that nurses can understand. Killick (2000) explained how the activity of storytelling remains essential for those with dementia, which threatens clients'

Box 11-2. Questions to Prompt Story Analysis

What values and beliefs are revealed in this story?

How does this person view life (as romance, comedy, or tragedy)?

What life themes emerge?

What parts of the story were given time, importance?

How does the past influence the present?

What unresolved conflicts are surfacing?

With what style is the story told?

For what might the story be a metaphor?

How distant (abstract) versus close to reality (concrete) is the story?

Why did the story get told now?

How is the protagonist (client) portrayed (as a martyr, warrior, victim, hero)?

Source: Taylor, E .J. (1995). The story behind the story: The use of storytelling in spiritual caregiving. *Seminars in Oncology Nursing, 13*(4), 252–254. Courtesy W. B. Saunders Co.

sense of self by interfering with the ability to know who they are and where they have been. Because of their threatened sense of self, it is vital that clients with dementia be encouraged to maintain a sense of identity through storytelling. Some may respond with irritation when a client's story seems confused. Killick's description of listening to the story of an elderly woman with dementia reflects a more appropriate attitude: "We are privileged to gain access to her mind, and for a few minutes see things as she sees them. Such a window into another's world is worth a dozen correct chronologies" (p. 10).

JOURNAL WRITING: REFLECTING THE SPIRIT

Keeping a journal or diary to privately chronicle life experiences is probably as old as writing itself. Journal writing nurtures the spirit by providing a medium by which clients can express their inner thoughts. This form of self-expression often increases self-awareness, central to spiritual awareness and development (see Chapter 3). Keeping such a chronicle also allows a client to learn from reviewing themes in his or her life and to take courage from recalling how past challenges were surmounted.

Journal Writing's Healing Effects

Although little empirical research exists that explores the effects of journal writing, acceptance of the practice as beneficial is widespread and long-standing. What evidence there is suggests that keeping a journal can assist adaptation to a traumatic event. In an experiment conducted by Pennebaker, Kiecolt-Glaser, and Glaser (1988), undergraduate students were asked to write for four days about either a superficial topic or a personal trauma they had experienced (e.g., leaving home and going to college, family problems, death of a loved one). Three months after the experiment, those who wrote about their trauma had significantly better immune function, had made fewer visits to the health center, and reported feeling happier than did the control group.

Journal writing can take many forms. Some clients may feel comfortable with the traditional diary or notebook. Others may want to chronicle their experiences in word documents that they file on a computer. Those who are intimidated by the process of writing may prefer to keep a "journal" by clipping meaningful quotes, stories, or pictures, or by jotting down thoughts on note cards and placing them in a special container.

The journal writer may want to consider the use of colored pens, pencils, or paper. The writing format can be as diverse as the form in which it is contained. Formats used in journal writing include:

- **Narratives** can be written about personal experiences, dreams, or fictional stories that express the spiritual desire. A narrative style can also be used to document an insight, record an interpretation, or give a status report on one's spirituality. One way to begin a journal entry is to choose a topic to explore (e.g., Who/what is God? What does forgiveness mean to me?)
- **Dialogues** can be written to describe an internal debate or conversation one is having with God, with society, with nature, with another individual, or with oneself or one's body part. A technique to try when creating a dialogue is to alternate the use of each hand. Writing the questions with the dominant hand and the answer (e.g., God's response or the obscured inner voice) with the nondominant hand is thought to allow the raw, unedited, authentic message to emerge.
- **Sketches** or **symbols** may be drawn to document spiritual responses or to depict objects or characters in a dream.
- **Mind mapping** or **clustering** is a way to capture ideas and concepts quickly and to link them with one another. Each idea is placed in a circle. Lines are drawn from each circle like spokes on a wheel to link concepts. This process encourages brainstorming and creativity.
- **Poetry** is a time-honored form of self-expression. Because spiritual journals are for the writers themselves to read, poetic self-expression does not have to follow any rules.
- **Prayers** may be entered in a journal to express lament, joy, desire, suffering, or other emotions. In a sense, many forms of journal writing are prayer.

Implications for Nursing Practice

When introducing a client to the process of journal writing, it is important to emphasize a few points. Unless they choose otherwise, their journal is for their eyes only. Thus, they need not be concerned about grammar or style and should refrain from judging their writing. Clients should consider journal writing a process rather than an outcome and anticipate that as with prayer, there may be dry times. Writing about an experience of spiritual drought can itself be spiritually nurturing. If someone feels an inner resistance to journal writing (or to prayer), examining it may support personal growth. The client can ask, "What am I avoiding? Why?" Finally, it is important to reread one's journal after which one may ask "What direction is my life taking?" or "What should be next for me?"

Other suggestions to launch the process of journal writing are found in Box 11-3.

Box 11-3. Ideas for Launching a Journal Entry

- Place your spiritual history on a timeline.
- Draw a symbol to represent your spirituality.
- Interview God, the Inner Wisdom, or yourself.
- Write lyrics for a song that describes something sacred.
- Describe and try to interpret a recent dream.
- Name a silent spiritual pain you experience. Describe it with seven adjectives or draw a sketch of it.
- Describe the people or events in your life that have influenced your spirituality.
- Respond to questions like:
  - How is God in my life today? This year? During my lifetime?
  - Where was the Ultimate Other when I experienced difficulty? Joy?
  - In what ways do I leave this world a better place?
  - What is sacred to me? How do I relate to that what is sacred?
  - In what ways do I resist becoming spiritually aware?
  - When/where do I feel "at home"—at peace, secure, joyful?
  - How does the way I feel physically influence how I am spiritually?
  - What role do feelings play in my being spiritually healthy?
  - Who am I? Where did I come from? Where am I going?

THE ARTS: EXPRESSING THE SPIRIT

Art is an expression of the soul (Samuels, 1995). This expression can take myriad forms: dance; visual arts (e.g., film, photography, drawing, sculpting, painting); music; crafts (e.g., weaving, sewing, pottery, carpentry, flower arranging); culinary art (e.g., baking, food sculpture and decorations); poetry and other literature; and so forth. Although art has become a commodity that is increasingly esteemed for its commercial value, its origins lie in religion and spirituality.

Steinhauser (1999) described a type of art as prayer (i.e., artprayer), a "communicative response of one's deepest being to a process initiated by God" (p. 13). Artprayer allows a whole-person (i.e., mind, body, and spirit) response to God, a contrast to the traditional experience of prayer as a conscious, cognitive process. This form of prayer affords self-expression in a concrete format. Steinhauser cautioned, however, that the focus of artprayer should remain on prayer, not the art itself. Self-expression via artwork, though spiritually edifying, is not artprayer.

How Art Nurtures the Spirit

Art aids spiritual healing in various ways (Bailey, 1997; Samuels, 1995). The act of creating art releases inner images that increase self-awareness. The use of an artistic medium to evoke order from chaos allows a client to make sense of experiences—a fundamental spiritual need. Creating art and sharing it with others allows clients to leave a legacy. When the act of creating art is a group endeavor (e.g., group singing or dancing), art serves to build a sense of community. An art object can aid spiritual healing by providing the viewer with a means for accessing mental images of healing. Art objects, like mandalas, icons, abstract sculpture, or landscape painting can also provide a focus for meditation.

Cassou and Cubley (1995), art therapists who describe painting as a way to "reclaim the magic of spontaneous expression," view painting as a process imbued with feeling. "To feel and to paint means to let the feeling sink deep into your bones, and then to start from that feeling without having to think about it" (p. 70). The desire to trash and restart a painting is a cue that a new feeling is emerging. Cassou and Cubley emphasize that creating art spontaneously without interpreting is essential to develop intuition and gain insight.

As with visual art forms, music also can soothe the spirit and become a means for focusing spiritual awareness. This is why, across cultures and denominations, music is an integral part of most religious worship services. Music's effect on the spirit may be indirectly evidenced by research that has demonstrated that music helps to decrease anxiety, depression, agitation, and aggressive behaviors; manage physical pain; and increase relaxation and positive mood (Cabrera & Lee, 2000; Snyder & Chlan, 1999). Music's powerful impact on human behavior is understood by many outside health care: Retail experts carefully select music for shopping venues and commercials to increase revenues; movie makers expertly craft music that accompanies film scenes to enhance viewers' emotional responses; and municipal managers choose music for subways and other public spaces that calms crowds.

Implications for Nursing Practice

Regardless of the preferred medium, clients will participate more readily in art making when they have access to materials of good quality. Because artistic inspiration can emerge at any time, these materials should be available to clients at all times. Drawing is an economical art form often used in clinical settings. An array of supplies should be provided (e.g., colored paper, chalk, pencils, paints, crayons).

To encourage clients to express themselves artistically, the nurse explores types of artistic expression that have been meaningful in the past. Although a client may prefer to repeat familiar methods, encouraging use of a new form may promote artistic expression without the interference of acquired skill. Creating a space for clients to display artwork may add meaning and beauty to a clinical setting. For some, however, artwork—especially artprayer—is a form of private expression. Steinhauser (1999) related how she deposited an artprayer to a place in the wilderness that seemed sacred.

Because nurses are not art therapists or psychotherapists, a few tips from experts may be helpful. Horovitz-Darby (1994) suggested that clinicians note a client's attitude toward and verbal commentary about the art, as well as its subject matter. Horovitz-Darby cautioned that asking a client to draw a picture of God can be offensive. Those who interpret literally the biblical commandment to refrain from making "any graven image" of God may object to this suggestion.

The nurse can introduce music to soothe and focus the client's spirit in a variety of ways. These include:

- Housing a small music library in a unit/department with portable, personal listening devices that can be loaned along with the tapes or compact discs.
- Organizing musicians (professional or amateur—even children) to provide mini-concerts in lobbies or other central locations in health care settings, or have them rove as minstrels.
- Playing inspirational music over public address systems at selected times.
- Singing or playing instruments (even kazoos!) with clients. Short, familiar secular (or if appropriate, religious) tunes will likely create the most successful performance and inspiriting effect.

Although many people think of inspirational music as slow-paced, religious, or melodic pieces of classical or "new age" genres, inspiration and spiritual focus can also come from listening to chants or upbeat, playful songs. When selecting inspirational music, the nurse elicits client preferences and endeavors to match them with spiritual needs.

To stimulate a client to undertake a visual art project, the nurse may offer ideas to which the client can respond in artistic form. Discussing the creation provides additional opportunities to promote client self-awareness. Box 11-4 provides tips for encouraging and evaluating this form of artistic expression.

Box 11-4. Facilitating Self-Expression with Art

To Stimulate Expression

Depict your spiritual home.

Draw your spiritual journey.

Draw how you relate with God, or Ultimate Other.

Illustrate your deepest desire.

Depict your spiritual feelings/state now (or, how your soul wants to speak now).

What would you create if you didn't have to worry about the way it looked?

(continues)

> **Box 11-4. Facilitating Self-Expression with Art *(continued)***

To Reflect upon Expression (Horovitz-Darby, 1994)

Please explain what you have created. What does it mean to you?

How did you experience the Divine while you created this art?

What feelings do you have about your art?

What in the creation process was joyful? Scary?

If you were a therapist, what interpretation would you give to this art?

DREAM WORK: WINDOWS TO THE SPIRIT

Dreams as well as visions and other paranormal experiences are prominent in many religious traditions. The Bible is replete with stories of people who experienced dreams, visions, or angelic visits (e.g., Abraham, Joseph, Daniel, and other Old Testament prophets; John, Peter, and other New Testament apostles). The emergence of some religions has been inspired by charismatic leaders who claimed to have had such experiences. Muhammad's visitation from angels, for example, led to the writing of the Koran and the beginnings of Islam. Likewise, William Smith's angelic visit from Moroni, the revelatory visions of Ellen White, Bah'u'llah, and Sun Myung Moon led to the founding of Mormonism, Seventh-day Adventism, Baha'i, and the Unification Church, respectively.

Within early Judeo-Christian religion, dreams were welcomed as an encounter with God and a gift for self-understanding (Savary, Berne, & Williams, 1984). Beginning around the fifth century C.E., mistranslation of the Bible, as well as Aristotelian and superstitious cultural influences, contributed to the disrepute of dreams in the Christian church and Western thought. This cynical and superstitious view of dreams has continued to the end of the twentieth century. A renewed interest in dreams, however, has emerged over the past quarter century or so, even Christian theologians and psychologists have reconsidered the divine gift of dreams.

What Are Dreams?

Nocturnal dreams have been defined as the "spontaneous symbolic experience lived out in the inner world during sleep" (Savary, Berne, & Williams, 1984, p. 4). O'Connor (1986) defined dreams as an avenue to the soul: "to dream is to make soul every night" (p. 63). Delaney (1993) identified several basic assumptions about dreaming that provide a conceptual basis for clinical applications:

- Dreams are expressions of feelings, thoughts, and ideas usually absent from the dreamer's waking awareness and that, when brought into that awareness, can enhance the dreamer's life.
- The effect of almost all recalled dreams is greatly enhanced by waking efforts to understand the dream in the context of the dreamer's life.
- Dreams have a point, a message intended to be grasped by the waking mind and used for the benefit of the dreamer.
- The dreamer, upon awakening, has all the information necessary to understand the dream.
- Dreams serve many functions. Dreams help us to process new information, correlate it with past experience, make sense of it, and learn from it. . . . Dreams express instinctual impulses, wishes, and defenses against them . . . [and] enable a dreamer to assess conflicts and resources (pp. 198–200).
- The cause and source of dreams are still unknown.

There are numerous types of dreams. In an editorial linking dreams with healing, Dossey (1999) provided examples of dreams that contain intimations of healing, wisdom, danger, death, disaster, and good fortune. Sanford (1968) distinguished among incidental personal dreams (what Freud called "day residues"), metaphoric dreams that impart personal and instructive meaning, and archetypal dreams that contain what Jung called "primordial images" that reflect the "collective unconscious."

Implications for Nursing Practice

Because nurses are not psychoanalysts or experts at dream analysis, their role in facilitating dream work is necessarily limited. Nurses can, however, encourage clients to respect and understand dreams. Thus, key elements of the nurse's role are to listen when a client wants to tell a dream and to educate clients about the value of dreams and techniques for understanding them. Several techniques suggested by experts on dreaming (e.g., Delaney, 1993; Guiley, 1995; Savary, Berne, & Williams, 1984) may be helpful:

- Some individuals believe that they rarely or never dream. Researchers, however, provide evidence that everybody dreams—

about fives times each night. Those who say they do not dream are unable to recall their dreams. Techniques for increasing dream recall include:

- Keeping a pencil and paper near one's bed and writing down the dream in a short hand manner before it is forgotten. (A penlight may be useful in the middle of the night.)
- Repeating an affirmation just before going to sleep such as "I will remember my dreams tonight."
- Upon awakening, resume the sleeping position and try to recall a dream.

- Recalling as many aspects of a dream as possible, verbally or in writing, is important. When recounting the dream, describe the sights, sounds, smells, and movements of each image in detail.
- Tell the dream story in first person in present tense (e.g., "I see someone approaching me . . ."). Any place in the recounting where the description reverts to past tense may indicate something from which the dreamer is distancing.
- The nurse should remain a curious listener during a client's dream telling. Interjecting observations or counter dream stories is unhelpful. Asking questions can facilitate a client's increased awareness of a dream and its meaning. When a client would benefit from prompting, helpful questions may include (Delaney, 1993):
  - What feelings are you most aware of in the dream? Do they remind you of anything in your current life?
  - Describe the opening of your dream. What type of place and mood did you experience? Does this remind you of anything?
  - Who is X (when a dream character is identified)? What kind of person is X? And what is X like in waking life? Does X remind you of anything in waking life? Such questions can also be framed to explore objects and actions in a dream.
- The TTAQ method for beginning to understand a dream has received wide use. This approach involves creating a title for the dream, identifying its theme and the affect(s) experienced during the dream, and asking what question the dream demands of the dreamer.
- Not until a dream has been completely recounted should the interpretation process commence. Begin simply by noting any immediate comments or reflections. Questions that encourage interpretation can be introduced, or questions the dreamer wants to ask of the dream may be given voice. In the process of understanding a dream, several

interpretations may be considered. Life events offer clues for dream interpretation as do themes from other dreams. Only the dreamer will know which interpretation fits. There will be an inner resonance or gut feeling when it is right.

- Engaging in dialogue with dream characters or images may afford insights. A dreamer can direct questions like "Why are you here?" or "What do you want to teach me?" to an image or character.
- Ultimately, spiritual development requires the dreamer to apply the lessons learned. The client can be encouraged to review a dream and its meaning a few times during the subsequent week. Failing to recall or enact the lessons of dreaming close this "avenue to the soul." (As with many things in life, "if you don't use it, you lose it.")
- It is possible that the meaning or lesson may be understood on some level during the dream. Action that draws on such insights can be applied should the dream reoccur (Fontaine, 2000). A menacing figure, for example, can be confronted with courage (rather than the initial fear) in subsequent dreams. Lessons drawn from acting with courage will be further understood with conscious dream analysis and can then be applied to life. Such responses often cause nightmares to diminish or cease.
- Although the mechanism is not well understood, some pharmaceuticals affect dreaming. Guiley (1995) noted that medicines used for treating cardiac conditions, hypertension, and Parkinson's disease can cause nightmares, as can fevers, surgery, and protein-rich foods. Recognizing that clients who take certain medications may be at risk for unsettling dreams encourages the nurse to offer emotional support.

Box 11-5 summarizes suggestions for facilitating dream work.

Box 11-5. Facilitating Dream Interpretation

Encourage clients to interpret their dreams by asking them to:
- Describe or write the dream with as much detail as possible using first person and present tense.
- Apply the TTAQ (i.e., Title, Theme, Affect, Question) technique.
- Respond to questions like the following:

(continues)

Box 11-5. Facilitating Dream Interpretation *(continued)*

- ○ How am I acting in the dream?
- ○ What feelings did I have during the dream? When have I felt this way in life?
- ○ Who or what is the adversary in the dream?
- ○ What would I like to avoid in the dream?
- ○ What symbols in the dream are important to me?
- ○ Does anything in this dream remind me of something or someone in my life?
- ○ What relation does the dream have to what is happening in my life right now?
- ○ Why did I need this dream?
- Choose an interpretation for which they have an intuitive "yes" that "clicks."
- Apply the lesson from their dreams to waking life.

Behaviors to avoid when clients recount their dreams:

- Don't put words in the dreamer's mouth or fill in the blanks (even if invited).
- Don't tell the dreamer how he or she felt.
- Don't encourage tangential discussions.
- Don't ask questions that are difficult to answer (e.g., "why?" or questions about forgotten aspects of the dream).
- Don't ask leading questions.
- Don't try to have the dreamer conclude an interpretation before fully describing the dream.
- Don't apply your metaphoric analysis or amplify their interpretation of the dream.
- Don't tell the dreamer what the dream means.

Sources: Delaney, G. (1993). The dream interview. In G. Delaney (Ed.), *New directions in dream interpretation* (pp. 195–240). Albany, NY: SUNY Press; Guiley, R. E. (1995). *The encyclopedia of dreams: Symbols and interpretations.* New York: Berkley Books; and Savary, L. M., Berne, P. H., & Williams, S. K. (1984). *Dreams and spiritual growth: A Judeo-Christian way of dreamwork.* Ramsey, N. J.: Paulist.

NURSING CONSIDERATIONS

An intriguing paradox often manifests when individuals consider an activity that fosters spiritual health. While people may recognize a need or desire to participate in a spiritual activity, they may also avoid participation. After the nurse introduces one of the activities discussed above to a receptive and eager client and provides concrete materials or guidance, the client may encounter barriers that discourage participation. Some may be superficial (e.g., "I don't have the time" or "I'm not good at that" or "I don't want anybody to see/hear the outcome"). Others may reflect deeper spiritual issues (e.g., "I'm afraid of what is inside me" or "I don't want to have to think about myself and face my realities"). An instinctive nursing response to superficial barriers is to protest and explain how to overcome them. These barriers, however, often reflect unexplored issues. A helpful nursing response is to allow the client to discover the deeper issue, a process that may defuse the barrier.

When introducing a spirit-nurturing activity, it is critical that the nurse approach the client with extreme sensitivity. Telling one's life story, sharing a dream, and expressing inner experience in an art form requires courage and results in vulnerability. Some clients may welcome a witness, a receptive listener, while others may choose to avoid vulnerability. The nurse respects client choices. Instead of sharing their spiritual experiences with the nurse, some clients will choose to share them with their clergy, family, or other confidante.

When a client chooses to share a story, dream, journal entry, or artwork, the nurse recognizes the client as the leader of ensuing dialogue. The client retains control about what is expressed and what meanings are ascribed to the experience. It is the client who ultimately knows the meaning of a story, dream, or artwork. A nurse, however, assists the client by asking reflective questions or serving as a silent, aware sounding board.

In the course of receiving a client's story, dream, or artwork, the nurse may sense that the client is experiencing spiritual or psychological distress that requires expert care. At such times, the nurse follows the guidelines offered in Chapter 8 for collaborating with spiritual care experts. A client, for example, may share a recurring dream that troubles him and express frustration with an inability to understand it. A referral to a psychoanalyst or pastoral counselor with expertise in dream analysis would be appropriate.

Self-disclosure is an important part of spirit-nurturing activities. Nurses may develop spiritual "therapy" groups in which clients implement these interventions. Storytelling, dream telling, and artwork have been used in client groups with a professional facilitator (Banks-Wallace, 1998; Cassou & Cubley, 1995; Dombeck, 1995). Groups that meet regularly provide a venue for self-disclosure and feedback from peers as well as social support.

Nurses may also enroll the services of trained volunteers. An avid gardener might receive satisfaction from assisting with the maintenance of flower boxes on a hospital unit and help clients to cultivate fast-growing plants. Pet owners and pets who are appropriately screened often love to provide "pet therapy" (Fontaine, 2000). Gifted listeners with some minimal training could assist with reminiscence therapy (Rybarczyk & Bellg, 1997). Artists of all kinds (e.g., dancers, painters, poets, musicians) can volunteer to provide their expertise.

The adage "See one, do one, teach one" applies to spirit-nurturing activities. Nurse educators have long known that students who can teach a peer to perform a nursing intervention are more likely to remember how to do it. A nurse who has kept a journal or a sketchpad or has experienced firsthand other nurturing activities brings added dimension to describing these activities to clients. Nurses, therefore, will benefit on many levels from exploring approaches to nurturing the spirit for themselves. Considering the nature of nursing work, the need of nurses for their own spiritual nurture is beyond question.

KEY POINTS

- Nature provides opportunities for self-awareness, peak experiences, and moments of transcendence. How one relates to nature may reveal much about how one relates to the Divine. Nature provides personal images of the Divine, as well as a medium and environment for meditation.
- Providing window views of natural surroundings and bringing pets, botanical life, or pictures of nature to clients are ways of exposing clients to nature's healing effects.
- Outcomes of storytelling include meaning making, self-understanding, and interpersonal connectedness.

- Strategies for facilitating spiritual growth through storytelling include helping clients to connect their stories to the present and to reframe them in a redeeming context, doing story checks, and sharing a counter story only when it would be therapeutic.
- Journal writing and creating art are methods for self-expression that increase self-awareness. There are numerous ways to approach these activities, and clients should be encouraged to follow their instincts without anxiety about "doing it right."
- Everyone dreams, and dreams are avenues to the soul. The role of the nurse is to listen when clients want to tell a dream, to educate clients about the value of dreams, and to offer techniques for understanding dreams.
- It is important for the nurse to consider the following points when introducing spirit-nurturing activities:
  - Address excuses or resistances, understanding that they often reflect deeper spiritual issues.
  - Respect the vulnerability involved in participating by allowing privacy. Encourage self-disclosure only when a client indicates the desire.
  - Allow the client to be the leader, controller, and interpreter; the nurse should function as a therapeutic listener.
  - Facilitate small group experiences for clients and involve volunteers with expertise in these spiritual activities.
  - Firsthand experience with these activities enhances the nurse's ability to facilitate them.

LOOK WITHIN TO LEARN

1. Imagine that you have been in a hospital or skilled nursing facility for three weeks and don't know when you'll be able to go home. You are finding it hard to "keep your spirits up." What would you want your nurse to do to help you boost your spirits? Would you like to experience nature? How? Would you like to tell your story and learn about yourself from the telling? Would you like to express yourself through art of some sort? How would you want your nurse to facilitate this for you? Is there anything else that might boost your spirits? How could a nurse help you with this?

2. Imagine having a chronic, disabling illness that prevents you from going out much. Your home care nurse explains how to keep a journal to chronicle your inner thoughts and feelings. You know that this would be a good idea, yet something stops you from starting. What barriers to keeping a journal might you (or other clients) encounter? Might these barriers apply to other activities that nurture your spirit? How might your nurse help you overcome these barriers?

REFERENCES

Bold print indicates those that are most recommended.

Bailey, S. S. (1997). The arts in spiritual care. *Seminars in Oncology Nursing, 13*, 242–247.
Banks-Wallace, J. (1998). Emancipatory potential of storytelling in a group. *Image: Journal of Nursing Scholarship, 30*, 17–21.
Brady, E. M. (1999). Stories at the hour of our death. *Home Healthcare Nurse, 17*, 176–180.
Brody, H. (1987). *Stories of sickness*. New Haven, CT: Yale University.
Cabrera, I. N., & Lee, M. H. (2000). Reducing noise pollution in the hospital setting by establishing a department of sound: A survey of recent research on the effects of noise and music in health care. *Preventive Medicine, 30*, 339–349.
Cassou, M., & Cubley, S. (1995). *Life, paint, and passion: Reclaiming the magic of spontaneous expression*. New York: Putnam.
Churchill, L. R., & Churchill, S. W. (1982). Storytelling in medical arenas: The art of self-determination. *Literature and Medicine, 1*, 73–79.
Cumes, D. (1998). Nature as medicine: The healing power of the wilderness. *Alternative Therapies in Health and Medicine, 4*(2), 79–85.

Delaney, G. (1993). The dream interview. In G. Delaney (Ed.), *New directions in dream interpretation* (pp. 195–240). Albany, NY: SUNY Press.

Dombeck, M. B. (1995). Dream telling: A means of spiritual awareness. *Holistic Nursing Practice, 9*(2), 37–47.

Dossey, L. (1999). Dreams and healing: Reclaiming a lost tradition. *Alternative Therapies in Health and Medicine, 5*(6), 12–17, 111–117.

Fontaine, K. L. (2000). *Healing practices: Alternative therapies for nursing.* Upper Saddle River, NJ: Prentice Hall.

Guiley, R. E. (1995). *The encyclopedia of dreams: Symbols and interpretations.* New York: Berkley Books.

Horovitz-Darby, E. G. (1994). *Spiritual art therapy: An alternative path.* Springfield, IL: Charles C Thomas.

Kelly, B. (1995). Storytelling: A way of connecting. *NursingConnections, 8*(4), 5–11.

Killick, J. (2000). Storytelling and dementia. *Elderly Care, 12*(2), 8–10.

Narayanasamy, A. (1995). Spiritual care of chronically ill patients. *Journal of Clinical Nursing, 4,* 397–398.

O'Connor, P. (1986). *Dreams and the search for meaning.* New York: Paulist Press.

Pennebaker, J. W., Kiecolt-Glaser, J. K., & Glaser, R. (1988). Disclosure of traumas and immune function: Health implications for psychotherapy. *Journal of Consulting and Clinical Psychology, 56,* 239–245.

Pickrel, J. (1989). "Tell me your story": Using life review in counseling the terminally ill. *Death Studies, 13,* 127–135.

Ruffing, J. (1997). "To have been one with the earth . . .": Nature in contemporary Christian mystical experience. *Presence: The Journal of Spiritual Directors International, 3*(1), 40–54.

Rybarczyk, B., & Bellg, A. (1997). *Listening to life stories: A new approach to stress intervention in health care.* New York: Springer.

Samuels, M. (1995). Art as a healing force. *Alternative Therapies in Health and Medicine, 1*(4), 38–40.

Sanford, J. A. (1968). *Dreams: God's forgotten language.* Philadelphia: Lippincott.

Savary, L. M., Berne, P. H., & Williams, S. K. (1984). Dreams and spiritual growth: A Judeo-Christian way of dreamwork. Ramsey, NJ: Paulist.

Snyder, M., & Chlan, L. (1999). Music therapy. *Annual Review of Nursing Research, 17,* 3–25.

Steinhauser, J. V. (1999). Artprayer: A dance with the holy. *Presence: The Journal of Spiritual Directors International, 5*(3), 8–17.

Taylor, E. J. (1997). The story behind the story: The use of storytelling in spiritual caregiving. *Seminars in Oncology Nursing, 13,* 252–254.

Travis, S. S., & McAuley, W. J. (1998). Mentally restorative experiences supporting rehabilitation of high functioning elders recovering from hip surgery. *Journal of Advanced Nursing, 27,* 977–985.

Index

Page numbers followed by f indicate figure.